POISON BY
PRESCRIPTION
The AZT Story

By John Lauritsen

Foreword by Peter Duesberg

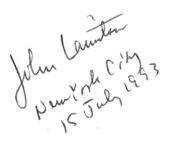

ASKLEPIOS
New York
1990

POISON BY PRESCRIPTION: The AZT Story
by John Lauritsen

Foreword by Peter Duesberg

Published by ASKLEPIOS/Pagan Press.

Fourth Printing: November 1992

Correspondence regarding this book should be directed to:
John Lauritsen, 26 St. Mark's Place, New York City 10003.

> *John Lauritsen's new book,* The
> AIDS War, *will be published by*
> *Asklepios early in 1993.*

If not available in a convenient bookstore, POISON BY
PRESCRIPTION can be ordered for $12 (postpaid) from the
author at the above address.

Library of Congress Catalog Card No. 90-81328
ISBN 0-943742-06-4

Dedicated to the "AIDS Dissidents" — who
dared to speak out during an epidemic of lies:

Jad Adams
Hansueli
  Albonico
Max Allen
Laurence Badgley
Michael
  Baumgartner
Harvey Bialy
Edward Brecher
Tony Brown
Frank
  Buianouckas
Allan Burns
Michael Callen
Mike Chapelle
Richard and
  Rosalind
  Chirimuuta
Seymour Cohen
Andrew Cort
Harris Coulter
Bryan Coyle
John Crewdson
Michael Culbert
Jon Damski
Luigi De Marchi
Brian Deer
Ola Deråker
James D'Eramo
Peter Duesberg
Eleni Eleopolis
Bryan Ellison
Michael Ellner
Celia Farber
Gene Fedorko
Giuliano Ferrieri
Fabio Franchi
Ron Gans
Ben Gardiner

Walter Gilbert
Cliff Goodman
Beverly Griffin
Group for the
  Scientific
  Reappraisal of
  the HIV-AIDS
  Hypothesis
H.E.A.L.
John Hammond
Albert Hässig
Nicky Hirsch
Neville
  Hodgkinson
Robert Hoffman
Bill and Claudia
  Holub
Drew Hopkins
Guido Hörner
Coleman Jones
Heinrich Kremer
Ilse Laas
Michael Lange
Robert Laarhovn
Nat Lehrman
Katie Leishman
Anthony
  Liversidge
Bruce Livesey
Cass Mann
Stuart Marshall
Clemmer
  Mayhew III
Patrick Merla
Kary Mullis
Roger Müller
Ehrhart Neubert
Gary Null
Luke Olmstead

Charles Ortleb
Neenyah Ostrom
Gérard Pollender
Positively Healthy
Projektgruppe
  AIDS-Kritik,
  Gesamtdeutsche
  Initiative
Jon Rappaport
Nick Regush
Robert Root-
  Bernstein
Harry Rubin
S.A.A.O.
  (Netherlands)
Ruth Sackman
Casper Schmidt
Peter Schmidt
Kawi Schneider
Russell Schoch
Craig
  Schoonmaker
Joseph Schwartz
Joan Shenton
Joseph
  Sonnabend
Tom Steele
Gordon Stewart
John Scythes
Michael Verney-
  Elliott
Erika Weiss
Hank Wilson
Michael Wilson
Ian Young

... and the many
others I may have
overlooked.

The Greek god of medicine, Asklepios, had two daughters who symbolized the two complementary aspects of the medical art: Panakeia symbolized the knowledge of drugs derived from the earth and from plants; Hygeia, the doctrine that the way to health is to avoid excesses and to live according to the laws of reason. (René Dubos, Man Adapting)

As the chill from the poison was reaching his groin, Socrates uncovered his face (for he had covered it) and said — they were his last words — "Crito, we should offer a cock to Asklepios. Will you remember?" "I will do it", said Crito; "Is there anything else?" There was no reply, and then the body moved. The attendant uncovered him. We saw that the eyes were set, and Crito closed the eyes and mouth.

And that, Echecrates, was the way our comrade died. I can honestly say, that of all the men I have known in our time, he was the bravest, and the wisest, and the most virtuous. (Plato, Phaedo)

CONTENTS

Foreword   7
Introduction   9

I.   POISON BY PRESCRIPTION: THE AZT STORY   11
II.   AZT ON TRIAL   25
III.   THE EPIDEMIOLOGY OF FEAR   48
IV.   ON THE AZT FRONT: PART ONE   59
V.   ON THE AZT FRONT: PART TWO   71
VI.   AZT AND CANCER   87
VII.   BURROUGHS WELLCOME ISSUES ADVISORY   104
VIII.   U.S. CUTS AZT DOSE IN HALF   114
IX.   AZT FOR HEALTHY PEOPLE   117
X.   A "STATE OF THE ART" AZT CONFERENCE   123
XI.   INTERVIEW WITH PETER DUESBERG (1987)   140
XII.   KANGAROO COURT ETIOLOGY   143
XIII.   INTERVIEW WITH PETER DUESBERG (1990)   169
XIV.   INCOMPETENCE IN AIDS EPIDEMIOLOGY   173

Appendix: New York Native Articles   184

Index   188

Illustrations
     Cover of New York Native, 1 June 1987   6
     Photograph of Peter Duesberg   142
     Photograph of Harry Rubin   150
     Photograph of fake slide   160
     Graph: AIDS Incidence By "Risk Groups"   176

N E W · Y O R K

NATIVE

Issue 215   June 1, 1987 $2.00

AZT

AZT is not a cure for AIDS.
AZT's alleged benefits are not
backed up by hard data, and are not
sufficient to compensate for the
drug's known toxicities.
Recovery from AIDS will come from
strengthening the body,
not poisoning it.
Do not take, prescribe, or
recommend AZT.
— *John Lauritsen (P. 14)*

Foreword

The DNA chain terminator AZT was designed over twenty years ago for the treatment of leukemia. Its antileukemic mechanism of action is to kill growing lymphocytes by termination of DNA synthesis. However, since AZT failed to prolong the lives of leukemic animals, it was not accepted for cancer chemotherapy. In 1987 it was approved to treat symptomatic and asymptomatic carriers of HIV to cure or prevent AIDS, based on the hypothesis that HIV causes AIDS. One year later, in 1988, the designers of AZT received a Nobel prize for medicine, although there was no evidence that AZT would cure or prevent AIDS.

The rationale of AZT therapy is simple, if not naive: the retrovirus HIV depends on DNA synthesis for multiplication, and AZT terminates DNA synthesis. Thus AZT should stop AIDS, if AIDS were caused by HIV, and if HIV were multiplying during AIDS. Yet there is still no proof for the now six year-old hypothesis that HIV causes AIDS. Moreover, many studies show that no more than one in 1,000 lymphocytes are ever infected by HIV -- even in people dying from AIDS. Since AZT cannot distinguish between an infected and an uninfected cell, 999 uninfected cells must be killed to kill just one HIV-infected cell. This means that AZT, as a treatment for AIDS, has a very high toxicity index. In view of this, there is no rational explanation of how AZT could be beneficial to AIDS patients, even if HIV were proven to cause AIDS.

There is always a small chance for an unpredictable effect, a miracle, even in science. If AZT were to prevent or cure AIDS despite the facts that the virus-AIDS hypothesis is ungrounded and that HIV does not make DNA during AIDS, it would be such a miracle. Unfortunately there is very little room for a miracle with AZT, because its mechanism of action is so embarrassingly clear, namely totally nonspecific termination of DNA synthesis. One could be lucky with miracle-anti-AIDS functions of drugs whose mechanism of action is poorly understood, such as aspirin, or even chicken soup -- but hardly with a substance that is a chain terminator of lymphocyte DNA synthesis in a person already deficient in lymphocytes.

It is conceivable that AZT may provide short-term benefits against AIDS to a person with acute microbial infections like tuberculosis, pneumonia, candidiasis or herpes, since these diseases are called AIDS if HIV antibody is present, by killing these microbes together with host cells. However, such infections could be controlled much better with confirmed, specific therapeutics than with the randomly toxic AZT.

The ultimate judge of a hypothesis like the virus-AIDS hypothesis is its usefulness in terms of therapeutic benefits and prevention. The virus-AIDS hypothesis has not stopped the spread of AIDS, it has not saved a single AIDS patient, and it is about to create 50,000 new ones -- the number of people currently being treated with AZT. Whatever slight claims AZT once had in being useful against AIDS -- have been "AZTed" by John Lauritsen's "Poison by Prescription: The AZT Story".

Peter Duesberg
Professor of Molecular Biology
University of California, Berkeley
April 1990

Introduction

The authoritarian mind-set of our times demands credentials. It is not enough to evaluate a man's argument on its merits: the quality of his evidence and reasoning. It is obligatory to know by what license, degree or title he has the authority to speak.

In writing these articles, I've tried to be both a good generalist and a good specialist. My academic background (Harvard) is in the social sciences, and I have two decades of experience as a survey research executive and analyst. Sometimes this background was helpful, as when analyzing clinical trials. But I've also had to study a number of fields that were new to me: medicine, molecular biology, public health, toxicology, etc. When necessary I've sought expert advice.

This book contains my major AZT articles from the New York Native, and some additional material. There is a certain amount of repetition, but I don't think a good reader will mind. In the midst of struggle, I have neither time nor energy to write an entirely new book. In addition, there may be historical value in preserving these articles as they were published.

Chapter I, "Poison By Prescription: The AZT Story", gives an overview of the situation as of about the middle of 1989.

Chapter II, "AZT On Trial", is the most important article -- an in-depth analysis of the Phase II trials, which were the basis of government approval for AZT, as well as claims that AZT "extends life".

Chapter III, "The Epidemiology of Fear", confronts bad government science exacerbated by bad journalism, laying to rest the claim that 99% of those infected with the "AIDS virus" will develop "AIDS".

Chapter IV describes dialogue on AZT among people with AIDS and physicians. Chapter V dissects a major AZT survival study, which has been used falsely to claim benefits for AZT.

Chapters VI through X describe chronologically the progress of a campaign to give AZT to healthy people. This unspeakably evil campaign, which I characterize as "iatrogenic genocide", is building momentum right now. The end result will be many tens of thousands of deaths from AZT poisoning -- deaths that predictably will be diagnosed and reported as "AIDS".

I have argued in print since 1984 that the "AIDS virus" is a poor candidate for causing "AIDS". In the summer of 1987 I was the first journalist to interview the molecular biologist, Peter Duesberg, and my interview with him in the Native was largely responsible for bringing the HIV debate into the public arena. Chapter XI is an excerpt from that interview, Chapter XII describes a forum where Professor Duesberg held his own against members of the "AIDS Establishment", and Chapter XIII is an excerpt from a more recent interview. Chapter XIV is a talk I gave at a Bronx forum, where every one of the speakers rejected the hypothesis that HIV is the cause of "AIDS".

I am proud to self-publish this book. In the absence of a free press -- and right now there is precious little free speech for "AIDS dissidents" -- I have done what had to be done, using the tools available to me. It's neither fun nor profitable to be the whistleblower on a dangerous drug. Anxiety is a constant companion, and friends and allies can seem few and far between. But my conscience is clear, and I am learning anew the value of self-reliance.

I hope to persuade the reader that I am right. The day is coming when historians will look back on the AZT episode as a tragedy, a crime against humanity, and one of the greatest frauds in medical history.

Sounding the tocsin on AZT is a job for all of us.

John Lauritsen
New York City
April 1990

I. Poison By Prescription:
The AZT Story

Tens of thousands of people are now taking a deadly drug which was approved by the United States government on the basis of fraudulent research. That drug is AZT, also known as Retrovir and zidovudine. It is the only federally approved drug for the treatment of "AIDS" (a poorly defined construct now encompassing more than two dozen old diseases).

AZT is not cheap. Treatment for a single patient costs between $8,000 and $12,000 per year, most of which is paid for, directly or indirectly, by taxpayer money.

The most toxic drug ever approved or even considered for long-term use, AZT is now being indiscriminately prescribed on a mass scale. Even the British manufacturer, Burroughs Wellcome, doesn't know for sure how many people are on AZT, but it may be as many as 50,000 worldwide. The great majority are gay men, but the drug is also being given to intravenous drug users, hemophiliacs and other people with "AIDS" (PWAs). Children, including new-born infants, are now receiving AZT, as are pregnant women who are "HIV-positive" (that is, who have antibodies to human immunodeficiency virus [HIV], which the world-renowned molecular biologist, Peter H. Duesberg, has described as a harmless and "profoundly conventional" retrovirus[1]). AZT is being given to healthy HIV-positive individuals, under the pretense that doing so will prevent "progression to AIDS". Some members of

---

[1]Peter H. Duesberg, "Human Immunodeficiency Virus And Acquired Immunodeficiency Syndrome: Correlation But Not Causation", Proceedings of the National Academy of Sciences, Vol. 86 (February 1989) pp. 755-764.

the "AIDS establishment", like William Haseltine (of the Harvard School of Public Health), have gone so far as to advocate giving AZT to perfectly healthy, HIV-negative members of "high risk groups", such as gay men, to prevent them from becoming "infected".

The prognosis cannot be not good for these people. AZT's toxicities are so great that about 50% of PWAs cannot tolerate it at all, and must be taken off the drug in order to save their lives. AZT is cytotoxic, meaning that it kills healthy cells in the body. AZT destroys bone marrow, causing life-threatening anemia. AZT causes severe headaches, nausea, and muscular pain; it causes muscles to waste away; it damages the kidneys, liver, and nerves. AZT blocks DNA synthesis, the very life process itself -- when DNA synthesis is blocked, new cells fail to develop, and the body inevitably begins to deteriorate.

The cumulative, long-term effects of AZT are unknown, since no one has taken the drug for more than three years. Even if patients were to survive the short-term toxicities of AZT, they would still face the prospect of cancer caused by the drug. According to the FDA analyst who reviewed the AZT toxicology data — and who recommended that AZT not be approved for marketing — AZT "induces a positive response in the cell transformation assay" and is therefore "presumed to be a potential carcinogen."[2]

Peter Duesberg has called AZT "pure poison".[3]

---

[2]Harvey I. Chernov, "Review & Evaluation of Pharmacology & Toxicology Data", NDA 19-655, 29 December 1986.   (FDA document obtained under the Freedom Of Information Act)

[3]John Lauritsen, "Saying No To HIV: An Interview With Prof. Peter Duesberg, Who Says, 'I Would Not Worry About Being Antibody Positive'; New York Na-

(continued...)

AIDS researcher and physician Joseph Sonnabend has stated that "AZT is incompatible with life".[4]

What benefits does AZT have, that could offset such terrible toxicities? None, as a matter of fact. AZT's benefits tend to vanish as soon as one scrutinizes them. The oft-repeated claim that AZT "extends life" is based on research that fully deserves to be called fraudulent.

The belief in AZT's benefits appears to be based on three bodies of "evidence". First are the Phase II ("Double-Blind, Placebo-Controlled") trials of AZT, conducted by the Food and Drug Administration (FDA). Second are anecdotal reports. Third is a report which has recently appeared in the Journal of the American Medical Association (JAMA). Let's look at these one at a time.

The Phase II Trials

(This section is based on documents that the FDA was forced to release under the Freedom of Information Act. A detailed analysis appears in my article, "AZT On Trial". Whitewashed reports on the Phase II trials can be found in two articles by Margaret Fischl and Douglas Richman in the New England Journal of Medicine.[5])

---

[3] (...continued)
tive, Issue 220, 6 July 1987; (Reprinted in Christopher Street, Issue 118, December 1987).

[4] John Lauritsen, "AZT: Iatrogenic Genocide", New York Native, Issue 258, 28 March 1988.

[5] Margaret A. Fischl, "The Efficacy of Azidothymidine (AZT) in the Treatment of Patients with AIDS and AIDS-Related Complex"; and Douglas A. Richman, "The Toxicity of Azidothymidine (AZT) in the Treat-
(continued...)

Phase I trials determined that it was possible to give AZT to human beings, although there was never any doubt that the drug was extremely toxic. The next step was the Phase II trials, conducted by the FDA at 12 medical centers throughout the United States, beginning in the spring of 1986. This "double-blind, placebo-controlled" study was designed so that two groups of "AIDS" patients would be "treated" for 24 weeks, one group receiving AZT and the other receiving a placebo. Neither the patients nor the doctors were supposed to know who was getting what.

In practice, the study became unblinded almost immediately. Some patients discovered a difference in taste between the AZT and the placebo capsules. Other patients took their capsules to chemists, who analyzed them. Doctors found out which patients were receiving AZT from very obvious differences in blood profiles. Thus, the very design of the study was violated. For this reason alone the Phase II trials were invalid.[6]

There are good reasons why blind studies are required for the approval of a new drug. The potential biases are so great, for both patient and doctor, that a drug-identified trial would be scientifically useless. Patients who believed that death was imminent without the intervention of a new "wonder drug", must have been psychologically devastated to learn that they were

---

[5](...continued)
ment of Patients with AIDS and AIDS-Related Complex", New England Journal of Medicine, 23 July 1987.

[6]Ellen C. Cooper, "Medical Officer Review of NDA 19-655". Additional evidence of the premature unblinding of the study comes from PWAs who participated in the Phase II trials and a chemist who analyzed the capsules, as featured on an NBC News (Channel 4) documentary, 27 January 1988.

only receiving a placebo. Physicians, with high expectations for AZT, may have been biased not only in the ways they interpreted and recorded data, but also in the way they treated their patients.   It is noteworthy that the public has never been informed by the FDA investigators, by Burroughs Wellcome, or by Fischl and Richman that the study became unblinded.

The FDA documents show that the Phase II trials were characterized throughout by sloppiness and lack of control. For example, recording forms for symptoms were so ineptly designed that the data had to be abandoned. Time and again the FDA documents suggest the likelihood of cheating. Case report forms were changed months after they had been recorded, with no explanations or indications of who had done the changing. Some of these changes favored AZT by reducing the cases of adverse reaction to the drug.[7]

At Boston, one of the twelve centers, an FDA investigator found serious problems: "multiple deviations from standard protocol procedure". She recommended that the Boston data be excluded from the study. In addition, numerous cases of "protocol violations" were discovered throughout the study. Most involved the unauthorized use of other drugs. The protocols were designed to prohibit multiple drug use, in order to avoid drug interactions and confounding the results.[8]

An FDA in-house meeting was convened to decide what to do about all of the bad data, the delinquent center, and the violations of protocol. The decision was made to keep everything. False data were retained. Garbage was thrown in with the good stuff. The researchers excused these inexcusable decisions on two grounds: One, if they didn't use the false data,

---

[7]Cooper, op. cit.

[8]Ellen C. Cooper, "Addendum #1 to Medical Officer Review of NDA 19-655", 16 March 1987.

there would be hardly any patients left in the study. Two, using the false data didn't really change the results very much. As every professional researcher knows, it is never acceptable to use false data. In and of itself, the deliberate use of false data made the Phase II trials not only invalid, but fraudulent.[9]

Midway through -- as the researchers were losing control and the study was bombing -- the trials were abruptly terminated. With much media fanfare it was claimed that AZT had miraculously preserved the lives of those taking it, and that it would therefore be 'unethical' to withhold AZT from PWAs, even for the few more weeks that would be required to carry the study through to completion. Allegedly only one patient on AZT had died, as opposed to nineteen patients on placebo, during an average treatment time of seventeen weeks. (As I'll argue later, these mortality claims are not to be believed.) At this point all patients were told whether they had been taking AZT or placebo (which many of them already knew) and were given the opportunity to take AZT.

The premature termination of the study destroyed the original study design, and caused chaos from an analytical standpoint. Twenty three of the patients had been 'treated' for less than four weeks; nevertheless, their data were thrown in along with everyone else's. Tables which would have been entirely straightforward if all patients had finished their 24 weeks of treatment had to rely upon weird statistical projections. For example, instead of showing the percentages of patients in each group who experienced opportunistic infections within 24 weeks, it became necessary to guess -- to develop a projected probability of their experiencing opportunistic infections within 24 weeks. This is analogous to estimating the probability of developing arthritis by the age of 70,

---

[9]Ibid.

using a sample in which only a few people had reached this age, and in which some were still children.[10]

In an Aesop Fable, a man boasts that, in an athletic competition on the island of Rhodes, he had performed a spectacular jump that no one could beat. Perhaps annoyed by his bragging, one of the men listening to him says: "Here is Rhodes. Jump here!" The principle applies in this case. If AZT could extend the lives of "AIDS" patients in the Phase II trials, then it could extend the lives of "AIDS" patients elsewhere. But the miracle has never repeated itself.

When the Phase II trials were over, most of the patients decided to begin or continue taking AZT. At this point the miracle was over. AZT didn't prevent them from dying. In 21 weeks 10% of the patients on AZT died (whereas allegedly less than 1% of the AZT patients had died during the miraculous 17-week treatment of the Phase II trials).

Another comparison: After the Phase II trials ended, AZT became available on a "compassionate plea" basis, and survival statistics were kept on 4,805 "AIDS" patients who took AZT. According to David Barry, Vice President in charge of research at Burroughs Wellcome, somewhere between 8% and 12% of the 4,805 "AIDS" patients treated with AZT died during four months (=17 weeks) of treatment.[11] In comparing the two groups -- each consisting of "AIDS" patients treated with AZT for 17 weeks -- we find an enormous difference: less than 1% died during the Phase II trials versus 8-12% (call it 10%) following release of the drug. (See table below.) A difference of this mag-

---

[10]Fischl and Richman, op. cit.; Lawrence Hauptman, "Statistical Review and Evaluation", NDA 19-655'; Ellen Cooper, "Medical Officer Review...".

[11]Telephone conversation with David Barry, 24 May 1988.

nitude cannot be due to chance -- the most likely explanation is that the less reliable figure (1%, from the Phase II trials) is wrong.

There are still more reasons for being skeptical of the mortality data from the Phase II trials.   The theory behind AZT is wrong: HIV (as argued persuasively by Duesberg and others) is not the cause of "AIDS".   And even if it were, a drug like AZT, designed to prevent the virus from replicating by stopping viral DNA synthesis, would be useless, since in "AIDS" patients HIV is consistently latent and therefore no longer making DNA.   On top of that, there is no evidence that AZT has any antiviral effect against HIV in the body, as opposed to the test tube.   (For awhile pro-AZT researchers were claiming results from the "P-24 antigen test", an unvalidated and highly inaccurate test, but such claims have been abandoned.)

MORTALITY COMPARISONS
(AIDS Patients Treated With AZT)

	Phase II Trials	Following Release Of Drug
Bases: Total Patients Treated With AZT In Each Trial	(145)	(4,805)
Deaths in 17 weeks	1%	10%*

* The probability is less than one in a million that the difference (1% vs. 10%) could be due to chance. This powerfully implies that the less reliable figure (1%) is wrong.

Still further grounds for skepticism concern the ethics and competence of the researchers. People who would knowingly tolerate cheating, who would use false data, and who would cover up the unblinding of a "double-blind" study, would be capable of other kinds of malfeasance. There are many unanswered questions on how Burroughs Wellcome received exclusive rights to AZT, and how this terribly toxic drug gained government approval faster than any drug in the FDA's history. The National Gay Rights Advocates (NGRA), has charged "illegal and improper collusion" between Burroughs Wellcome and two federal agencies, the National Institutes of Health (NIH) and the FDA. Shortly after Burroughs Wellcome sent a check for $55,000 to Samuel Broder of the National Cancer Institute (part of the NIH), Burroughs Wellcome received exclusive rights to market AZT, even though AZT had been in existence for 20 years and Burroughs Wellcome had played no part in the drug's development.[12]

Finally, the Phase II mortality data are suspect because the researchers performed no autopsies on the patients who died, and released almost no information on the causes of death. The FDA refuses even to divulge what cities the patients died in.

Summing up: It is highly unlikely that AZT extended the lives of patients in the Phase II trials. There are at least three explanations, not mutually exclusive, to account for the alleged mortality data. One, since the study became unblinded and the doctors knew which patients were receiving each treatment, the AZT patients, unconsciously or deliberately, may have received better patient management; the placebo patients may have been killed off through neglect. Two, the sicker

---

[12]Ray O'Loughlin, "Lawsuit Charges Collusion Between Feds, AZT Maker", Bay Area Reporter, 5 November 1987.

patients may have been placed in the placebo group to begin with. (The FDA documents indicate that this was indeed the case.[13]) <u>Three</u>, there may have been deliberate cheating: some dead AZT patients may have been posthumously reassigned to the placebo group. Given the sloppiness of the trials, and the deplorable standards of the researchers, the third explanation is entirely plausible.

Aside from the doubtful mortality data, there is the issue of AZT's toxicities. The FDA analyst who reviewed the pharmacology data, Harvey I. Chernov, recommended that AZT should <u>not</u> be approved. Chernov documented many serious side effects of AZT, and summarized its effect on the blood as follows: "Thus, although the dose varied, anemia was noted in all species (including man) in which the drug has been tested."[14]

Anecdotal Reports

At the Stockholm "AIDS" conference last summer a number of abstracts were presented, which claimed various benefits for AZT. These abstracts consisted of unpublished data derived from uncontrolled observations of small numbers of patients. For scientific debate, the value of such reports, in the context of a conference where 3200 abstracts were presented, is nil. Such abstracts amount to little more than anecdotal evidence.

One of the more absurd abstracts was later pub-

---

[13]Cooper, <u>Medical Officer Review...</u>".

[14]Harvey I. Chernov, "Review & Evaluation of Pharmacology & Toxicology Data".

lished in the New England Journal of Medicine[15]. Researchers connected with the government and Burroughs Wellcome gave AZT to 21 children who had "HIV infection", and claimed that the AZT boosted their IQs by 15 points. Although 5 of the 21 children died, the researchers were so impressed by "neurodevelopmental" improvements that they recommended giving AZT to "infected but asymptomatic newborns". Anyone who has studied the principles and techniques of psychological testing can only have contempt for this misuse of intelligence tests.

Another variety of anecdotal report comes from physicians who treat "AIDS" patients. These doctors, many of them rather gullible individuals, have been told that AZT represents the "best hope". With this expectation, they begin dosing their patients with AZT, and sooner or later some of them believe that they have "seen good results". Of course, "good results" may not be good by any rational criteria. Perhaps a patient, having undergone multiple transfusions and suffered agonizing side effects, dies after 11 months; the doctor can then rationalize that he would have died sooner if it hadn't been for the AZT. Doctors in New York City have begun experimenting with reduced doses of AZT (half doses, quarter doses, or even less), as well as AZT in combination with many other drugs. Experimentation of this sort, with no sound basis in either theory or fact, is no better than the use of frog skins, leeches, crystals and the like.

For every doctor who has "seen good results", there may well be ten doctors who have seen bad results. As the latter observations are not fashionable, they are

---

[15]Philip A. Pizzo, et al., "Effect of Continuous Intravenous Infusion of Zidovudine (AZT) in Children with Symptomatic HIV Infection", New England Journal of Medicine, 6 October 1988.

not likely to find expression in abstracts at "AIDS" conferences.

The JAMA Article

A major study of AZT, "Survival Experience Among Patients With AIDS Receiving Zidovudine [AZT]", recently appeared in the Journal of the American Medical Association (JAMA).[16]   AZT promoters have used this study to claim that AZT extends the lives of PWAs.

Researchers from the government and Burroughs Wellcome studied 4,805 PWAs treated with AZT. Through colossal incompetence they lost track of 1120 patients, not knowing if they were even alive or dead. The researchers then used statistical projection methods to guess what results they might have obtained if they had not lost the 1120 patients, and came up with a 10-month survival estimate of 73%. They then wrote their report in such a way that the 73% guess appeared to be an actual survival statistic. Finally, they made a number of grossly invalid comparisons to other groups of PWAs, unjustifiably claiming that AZT had extended the lives of those in their study.

It is a sad commentary on the standards of medical journals that JAMA would publish this blatant exercise in disinformation.

The AZT Philosophy

The question arises: How can physicians justify prescribing a drug whose benefits are so dubious and whose side effects are so terrible? Physicians are supposed to honor the Oath of Hippocrates, the car-

---

[16]Terri Creagh-Kirk et al., "Survival Experience Among Patients With AIDS Receiving Zidovudine [AZT]: Follow-up of Patients in a Compassionate Plea Program", Journal of the American Medical Association, 25 November 1988.

dinal principle of which is to act for the good of the patient, doing nothing that is harmful.

There seem to be two pillars to the AZT philosophy. First is the American faith in drugs as the appropriate treatment for almost everything. The more potent and expensive the drug, the better.

Second is the prevailing belief that "AIDS" is "invariably fatal", that PWAs have only a few months to live. For example, the JAMA article discussed above asserts, "AIDS is a terminal disease". Physicians who accept this premise can simply ignore the cumulative toxicities of AZT.

There are several objections to the AZT philosophy. Most important, "AIDS" is not invariably fatal. There are PWAs who have survived for many years, and who appear to be recovering. And why not? What other disease is "invariably fatal"? I imagine that future medical historians will regard many or even most of the "AIDS" fatalities as iatrogenic: caused by medical treatments rather than by "AIDS" itself. The sick deserve a chance to recover. With AZT there is little chance.

A Philosophy For Recovery

To be honest, at this point we do not know exactly what "AIDS" is, or what causes it, or how to treat it (although physicians are getting better at treating the various opportunistic infections). From all of the evidence, it appears unlikely that "AIDS" is a single disease entity caused by a novel infectious agent, HIV or other. Rather, "AIDS" appears to be a condition or conditions which may arise from multiple causes. In my opinion, chemicals (including recreational drugs, antibiotics, and medical drugs) probably play the primary role in making gay men and intravenous drug users sick, but that is another discussion.[17]

If "AIDS" is really a degenerative condition caused largely by toxins, both medical and "recreational", then what is an appropriate treatment?   Not still another drug, but rather freedom from toxins.   Long-term survivors, almost without exception, have avoided toxic chemotherapy (like AZT) and have opted for repairing their bodies through a more healthy lifestyle: exercise, good nutrition, rest and stress reduction, and avoidance of harmful substances (including cigarettes, alcohol, heroin, cocaine, MDA, quaaludes, barbiturates, Eve, Ecstasy, PCP, TCP, Special K, ethyl chloride, poppers, and all other "recreational drugs").

Human bodies are the product of millions of years of evolution, in a universe filled with microbes of all kinds; if allowed to, they know how to heal themselves.   Recovery from "AIDS" will come from strengthening the body, not poisoning it.

#

---

[17]John Lauritsen, "CDC's Tables Obscure AIDS-Drugs Connection", Philadelphia Gay News, 14 February 1985.   Also many articles in the New York Native from 1985 to the present.

John Lauritsen and Hank Wilson, Death Rush: Poppers & AIDS, New York, 1986.

II. AZT On Trial

I argued in a previous article ("First Things First") that the theory behind AZT (now known by its trade name of Retrovir) was false, inasmuch as the hypothesis that HIV causes AIDS has been refuted by Prof. Peter H. Duesberg, a world-renowned molecular biologist at Berkeley[1]; that AZT's alleged benefits were not backed up by reliable evidence; that its toxicities were firmly established and severe; and therefore the drug should not be prescribed, recommended, or used.

In his interview with me[2], Prof. Duesberg referred to AZT as "a poison" and as "cytotoxic" (lethal to body cells). Duesberg said that the theories behind AZT were false, that there was "no rationale for treating with AZT", that prescribing AZT was "highly irresponsible", and that AZT was "guaranteed" to be harmful:

AZT hits all DNA that is made. It is hell for the bone marrow, which is where the T and B cells and all those things are made. It's hell for that. It has a slight preference for viral DNA polymerase compared to cellular DNA polymerase, based on in vitro studies only, but that's certainly not absolute. It kills normal cells quite, quite extensively.[3]

---

[1]Peter H. Duesberg, Ph.D; "Retroviruses as Carcinogens and Pathogens: Expectations and Reality"; Cancer Research; 1 March 1987.

John Lauritsen, "Saying No to HIV: An Interview With Prof. Peter Duesberg", Native, Issue #220.

[2]Lauritsen and Duesberg, op. cit.

[3]Ibid.

At the time these articles were published, the only reports on the Food and Drug Administration (FDA) trial that was the basis for granting government approval to market AZT, were in the popular media or a promotional film produced by AZT's manufacturer, Burroughs-Wellcome. Doctors who prescribed AZT did so on the basis on very limited information, along with the assurances of the Public Health Service that AZT represented the "best hope".

This appears to have changed. The 23 July 1987 issue of the New England Journal of Medicine (NEJM) contains a two-part report on the FDA's "Double-Blind, Placebo-Controlled Trial"[4]

It quickly became clear to me that there were serious problems with the reports. The description of methodology was incomplete and incoherent. Not a single table was acceptable according to statistical standards -- indeed, not a single table made sense. In particular, the first report, on "efficacy", was marred by contradictions, ill-logic, and special pleading.

In the meantime, I received about 500 pages of material which Project Inform in San Francisco had obtained from the FDA under the Freedom of Information Act. This material showed the dark underside of the double-blind, placebo-controlled trial -- falsification of data, sloppiness, confusion, lack of control, departure from accepted procedures -- things not even hinted at in the NEJM reports. Martin Delaney of Project Inform gives a fair summary of what emerges from the FDA material:

---

[4]Margaret A. Fischl, M.D.,"The Efficacy of Azidothymidine (AZT) in the Treatment of Patients with AIDS and AIDS -Related Complex"; and Douglas D. Richman, M.D.,"The Toxicity of Azidothymidine (AZT) in the Treatment of Patients with AIDS and AIDS-Related Complex"; New England Journal of Medicine, 23 July 1987.

The multi-center clinical trials of AZT are perhaps the sloppiest and most poorly controlled trials ever to serve as the basis for an FDA drug licensing approval. Conclusions of efficacy were based on an endpoint (mortality) not initially planned or formally followed in the study after the drug failed to demonstrate efficacy on all the originally intended endpoints. Because mortality was not an intended endpoint, causes of death were never verified. Despite this, and a frightening record of toxicity, the FDA approved AZT in record time, granting a treatment IND in less than five days and full pharmaceutical licensing in less than 6 months.

After reading through the FDA material several times, I called Margaret Fischl and Douglas Richman, the primary authors of the NEJM articles, and spoke with each of them for about half an hour. The conversations were not very enjoyable for any of us. Neither one of them could explain the tables in the reports that they themselves had supposedly written. They both repeatedly said that I should call Burroughs-Wellcome to find out how the tables were developed or to obtain answers on other questions. Richman became quite truculent at one point, saying that I was "fixated" on the tables; that I should "forget about the tables"; that the report would be "just as good without them". Their ignorance regarding these tables is really amazing. As a market research analyst, I am accustomed to working with tables, and I can say that I have never written a report containing even a single table I could not explain and interpret.

Despite abundant reports of the horrible physical consequences of taking AZT, several of the New York City physicians most prominent in treating AIDS and ARC patients are not only prescribing AZT, but actively proselytizing for it. I think that history will judge these doctors harshly. This article will argue that no credence should be placed in the NEJM reports, that the "benefits" attributed to AZT remain unsubstantiated.

The aborted trial

The "double-blind, placebo-controlled" trial of AZT was conducted by the FDA at twelve medical centers throughout the United States. Although the patients did not enter the study all at one time, each patient was intended to undergo a full 24 weeks of "treatment" — either with AZT or with a placebo.

Midway through the study it was observed that only one patient on AZT had died, whereas more than a dozen on placebo had. According to the received version, the FDA then decided it would be unethical to continue the study, since AZT was so spectacularly (if unexpectedly) prolonging the lives of those who took it. The study was terminated; all patients were told whether they had been taking AZT or a placebo, and all were given the opportunity to take AZT. As I'll argue later, there are good reasons for being skeptical of the mortality data, as well as the motives for prematurely terminating the study.

Owing to the early termination, only 15 patients (5% of the total) completed the full 24 weeks of treatment. Twenty-three patients were treated for less than four weeks. On the average, patients had received treatment for about 17 weeks at the time the study was aborted. (See Table 1.)

As might be imagined, the premature termination invalidated the original study design and caused chaos from an analytical standpoint. Tables which would have been entirely straightforward if all patients had finished their 24 weeks of treatment had to rely upon controversial statistical projections. For example, instead of showing the percentages of patients in each group who experienced opportunistic infections during the 24 weeks, it became necessary to develop a projected probability of their experiencing opportunistic infections within 24 weeks. This is analogous to estimating the probability of developing arthritis by the age of 70, using a sample in which only a few people had reached this age, and in which some were still teenagers. The method used (Kaplan-Meier Product-Limit Method) is a statistical attempt to estimate what results would have been if the study had not been terminated. Like mopping up milk, it may be the best thing to do -- but it would be better not to spill the milk.

TABLE 1

VERY FEW PATIENTS FINISHED THE FULL 24-WEEK PROTOCOL

	Total Patients	Treatment AZT	Placebo
Base: Total Who Began Trial	(282)	(145)	(137)
Finished Trial	5%	6%	4%
Did Not Finish Trial	95%	94%	96%
"Still Participating"	73%	79%	67%
Dropped Out of Study	22%	15%	29%
Weeks of Treatment (Mean)	(17.3)	(17.6)	(16.9)

[NOTE: ALL TABLES IN THIS ARTICLE ARE MY OWN; THEY ARE NOT TAKEN FROM THE NEJM REPORTS.]

With poignant restraint, an FDA mathematical statistician registered his misgivings over the early termination:
There are a number of disquieting aspects concerning this NDA. It contains only one con-

trolled clinical trial, and thus there is no in-
dependent confirmatory evidence for that study's
results. It contains a relatively small number of
patients (<200) who have been treated with AZT.
The controlled clinical study is relatively short
(i.e., 24 weeks) and was terminated early on the
basis of unanticipated favorable results in a
manner that has never been adequately defined
in terms of its impact on the subsequent statistical analyses.[5]   [Emphasis added.]

The unblinded trial

The study was planned as a "double-blind" trial,
which means that the drug was supposed to be labelled
and the study conducted in such a way that neither
doctors nor patients knew whether AZT or a placebo
was being administered.

In practice, the AZT trial became unblinded rather
quickly. An FDA medical officer writes: "the fact that
the treatment groups unblinded themselves early could
have resulted in bias in the workup of patients".[6]

The study became unblinded among the patients as a
result of differences in taste between AZT and the
placebo:

Initially the placebo capsules, which were indis-
tinguishable from the AZT capsules in ap-
pearance, were distinguishable in taste. This
difference was corrected and the placebo capsules replaced with new ones after early reports

---

[5]Lawrence Hauptman, Ph.D.; "Statistical Review
and Evaluation"; NDA# 19-655/Drug Class 1A,
Burroughs-Wellcome Company, AZT Capsules; p. 17.

[6]Ellen C. Cooper, M.D., M.P.H.; "Medical Officer
Review of NDA 19-655"; p. 70.

were received of patients breaking the capsules and tasting the medication.[7]

Anyone who has spent time with PWAs is aware of the keen interest with which they compare treatments. And anyone who has observed the gay grapevine is in awe of the speed with which information can travel around the world. I can well believe that from the time the first two patients compared notes on how their capsules tasted, it was only a matter of days until many or most of the patients knew whether they were getting AZT or a placebo.

Other patients discovered what medication they were receiving by taking their capsules to chemists for analysis.

In some instances patients pooled and shared their medication, thus ensuring that all of them could receive at least some AZT. Other patients, who found out their medication was only a placebo, took Ribavirin that had been smuggled in from Mexico.

From the standpoint of the doctors, the study unblinded itself through the strikingly different blood profiles of the two treatment groups. (See "Toxicity" below.) No attempt was made to blind the blood results from any of the doctors in the medical centers at which the trials were held. According to an FDA analyst:

> The treatment groups may have unblinded themselves to a large extent during the first two months due to drug-induced erythrocyte macrocytosis.[8]

There are very good reasons why blind studies are required for the approval of a new drug. The poten-

---

[7]Ibid. p. 6.

[8]Ibid. p. 70.

tial biases are so great, for both patient and doctor, that a drug-identified trial would be scientifically useless.

Many patients entered the trial believing that death was immanent without the intervention of a new "wonder drug". For these patients, the psychological consequences of finding out that they were receiving only a placebo must have been devastating. A sense of despair and hopelessness may well have contributed to the high mortality in the placebo group.

Doctors, and scientists in general, are often extremely gullible people. In their book, Betrayers of the Truth: Fraud and Deceit in the Halls of Science, William Broad and Nicholas Wade devote an entire chapter to "Self-Deception and Gullibility". Scientists unconsciously see what they want to see. Even the most absurdly crude hoaxes, like the Piltdown man, were believed for many years by eminent scientists. With high expectations engendered for AZT, it is not unreasonable to assume that unconscious biases affected not only how data were interpreted and recorded, but also how patients were treated. The shockingly high death rate among the placebo patients suggests that these patients may not have been managed well by their attending physicians.

When I spoke to Fischl and Richman, they both vehemently denied that the trial had become unblinded before it was terminated. This suggests that they had little control over, or knowledge of, what was happening -- or, that they were not telling the truth. As FDA analyst Cooper stated, it was fact that the study became unblinded early on. And since the AZT trial was not blinded, the entire study was invalid and worthless. On this basis alone, FDA approval of the drug was neither proper nor legal.

Sloppiness, improprieties, false data

The AZT trial was characterized throughout by sloppiness and lack of control. Recording forms were poorly designed, leading to confusion when doctors were asked to make judgments. For example, doctors were asked to record 10 subjective symptoms "often associated with HIV infection", and to decide whether they were symptoms of AIDS or adverse reactions to the drug treatment. Understandably it was hard to differentiate among "malaise, fatigue, and lethargy", let alone to decide whether these were caused by drug or by disease. Midway through the trial the "sponsor" (Burroughs-Wellcome) substituted a 33-item "AIDS-related signs and symptoms" sheet, at which point confusion became utter chaos. Most of the medical centers were unable to relate one form to the other, or even to comprehend the 33-item form, and so in the end the incomplete data on the 10-item form served as the patients' only baseline data.

When FDA analysts reviewed the Case Report Forms, numerous improprieties were observed:

Symptoms previously checked off on the 10-item sheet were crossed out or otherwise changed, usually without the principal investigator's initials, and sometimes with a date of change much later than the date the form was originally filled out, without explanation as to why changes were made.

"Transcription" of data from 10-item symptom form to the 33-item form was performed, sometimes without date of initials of who did the transcribing. Sometimes the original form was not submitted.

Adverse experiences were sometimes crossed out months after initially recorded, even though "possibly related to test agent" had been checked off originally by the investigator or his designee.[9]

The last set of improprieties is especially serious, as it appears to be tendentious, favoring AZT by reducing the cases of adverse reactions to the drug. If done deliberately this would constitute cheating and fraud, things that people supervising studies must constantly be vigilant against. If there can be cheating in little things, there can be cheating in big things as well.

Having detailed these various improprieties, the FDA analyst insouciantly dismissed the whole mess with a sentence that caught me completely off guard:

Whatever the "real" data may be, clearly patients in this study, both on AZT and placebo, reported many disease symptom/possible adverse drug experiences.[10]

"Whatever the 'real' data may be..."! I can't get over this phrase. Is this an expression of bureaucratic cynicism, a sardonic form of humor, or what? Do FDA analysts even care whether their data is "real" or not?

Serious problems were uncovered at one of the 12 medical centers. According to an FDA analyst:

The FDA inspector found multiple deviations from standard protocol procedure, and she recommended that data from this center be excluded from the analysis of the multicenter trial. [Emphasis added.][11]

---

[9]Ibid. pp. 77-78.

[10]Ibid. p. 78.

[11]Ellen C. Cooper, M.D.; "Addendum #1 to Medical Officer Review of NDA 19,655; p. 1.

The FDA inspector's report did not reach an appropriate department until late December 1986, three months after the trial had been terminated. The decision was then made...

> to request inspection of all twelve centers which participated in this trial, due to the importance of this drug, its high public visibility, and because one of the early inspections had revealed "significant deviations" from FDA regulations regarding the proper conduct of clinical investigations.[12]

At this point inspecting all 12 centers was like locking the barn after the horse was stolen. Of grave concern is the fact that one of the problems noted in the delinquent center had to do with "drug accountability", perhaps the most serious impropriety that could be imagined. If there is even the slightest doubt that all "AZT patients" really were getting AZT, and all "placebo patients" really were getting placebos, then the study has fallen apart at its very core.

In addition, there were numerous cases of "protocol violations". When the study was designed, various conditions were defined as constituting "protocol violations", as a result of which a patient's data would be excluded from the data base. Most of the protocol violations concerned the unauthorized use of other drugs in addition to the treatments administered in the study. These restrictions were necessary in order to avoid drug interactions, confounding results, and so on. At an FDA in-house meeting convened to decide what to do about the patients in whom protocol violations were noted, one FDA officer commented that "if exclusion of all patients with protocol violations were

---

[12]Ibid. p. 1.

strictly applied, quite a few patients would probably be deleted from the database."[13]

After agonizing over the "highly visible, potentially inflammatory issue" of whether to exclude data from the delinquent center or from patients with protocol violations, it was decided to exclude nothing.   False data were retained.   Garbage was thrown in with the good stuff.   This was the rationalization:

> Because the mortality analyses were so strongly in favor on the drug, any slight biases that may have been introduced when minor 'protocol' violations occurred were highly unlikely to influence the outcome."[14]

This is egregiously beside the point.   It is irrelevant whether or not throwing in bad data with good data will "influence the outcome".   The point is that you don't do it on principle.   It is an absolute and iron-clad principle of research that you don't use bad data.   No principled analyst would ever proceed to interpret data that he knew were contaminated.   One may note that not a hint of these problems appears in the NEJM reports by Fischl and Richman.

Mortality

The mortality data that so dazzled the FDA that they terminated the AZT trial prematurely and accepted bad data are shown in Table 2.   Only 1% of the 145 AZT patients, compared to 14% of the 137 placebo patients died during the course of the trial.   Statistically, this is highly significant — the probabilities are better than 99 out of 100 that the difference (1% vs. 14%) is real, as opposed to being a product of chance.

---

[13]Ibid. p. 2.

[14]Ibid. p. 3.

TABLE 2

MORTALITY
DOUBLE-BLIND, PLACEBO-CONTROLLED TRIAL

	Treatment	
	AZT	Placebo
Base: Total Who Began Trial	(145)	(137)
Cumulative Deaths During Trial	1%	14%*
Weeks Of Treatment (Mean)	(17.6)	(16.9)

*Significantly higher than AZT at the 99% confidence level.

_____

One must caution, however, that these mortality data reflect a very short time period -- only 17 weeks, on the average. It would be fallacious to assume that the death rate would have continued to be higher in the placebo group if the time period were 30 weeks, or a year, or two years.

In addition, there are good reasons to be skeptical of the mortality data. For one thing, the death rate in the placebo group is shockingly high. According to doctors in New York with extensive experience in treating AIDS patients, with good patient management, nowhere near this many patients ought to have died in such a short time.

In addition, the death rate in the AZT group is suspiciously low when compared with other trials of AZT. After the "double-blind, placebo-controlled" study was terminated, all patients were informed which treatment they had been receiving, and were offered the option of receiving AZT. (See Table 3) A total of 227 patients accepted the offer, and continued or began to receive AZT (127 who were originally treated with AZT and 100 who were originally treated with placebo). AZT no longer prevented patients from dying. In the 21 weeks of the "open-label" trial, 10% of the patients died. Curiously, not only deaths but also opportunistic infections increased in the original AZT group as soon as the first study was terminated. There is no good explanation why this should be so.

TABLE 3

MORTALITY

OPEN-LABEL TRIAL FOLLOWING TERMINATION
OF DOUBLE-BLIND, PLACEBO-CONTROLLED TRIAL
(18 September 1986 - 13 February 1987)

	Total Patients	Treatment	
		AZT	Placebo
Base: Total Participating	(227)	(127)	(100)
Cumulative Deaths During Open-Label Trial (21 Weeks Of Treatment)	10%	8%	12%

Another trial of AZT occurred prior to the "double-blind, placebo-controlled" trial. (See Table 4) This was a "Phase I" trial, intended to give a preliminary estimate of the drug's toxicities. In the Phase I trial, 12% died during a time period of only 6 weeks. The four patients who died were replaced, and all 33 patients continued to take AZT in an "extended trial", during which an additional 21% died. It is unclear from the FDA material exactly how long the extended trial lasted — but at any rate a cumulative total of one-third (33%) of the patients died, either in the phase I or in the extended trial.

Burroughs-Wellcome provided data to the FDA on deaths which occurred among patients who began taking AZT following release of the drug. The information was in incredibly garbled form, but I was able to ascertain at least the deaths that occurred during the first 8 weeks of treatment. During this short time period 6% of the patients died.

TABLE 4

MORTALITY

PHASE I TRIAL OF AZT
(No Placebo Control)

Base: Total Receiving AZT	(33)
Deaths During 6-Week Trial	12%
Deaths During Extended Trial	21%
Cumulative Deaths	33%

Table 5 shows a comparison of these four studies of AIDS or advanced ARC patients who were treated with AZT. It can readily be seen that the death rate in the "double-blind, placebo-controlled" trial (the first column) is significantly lower than in any of the other studies, especially considering that the trials in columns three and four represented much shorter time periods. In other words, the mortality data from the "double-blind, placebo-controlled" trial are almost certainly wrong, based on comparisons with mortality data from other AZT trials.

In addition, skepticism is warranted by virtue of the stakes involved, hundreds of millions of dollars. The materials released by the FDA show that both the FDA and Burroughs-Wellcome were quite willing to bend rules if doing so would facilitate approval for AZT.

The FDA did not come to the AZT trials with clean hands. In fact, the FDA has a long history of collusion with industry. A number of examples can be found in the book, How to Get Rid of the Poisons in Your Body, by Gary Null and Steven Null.

Another example where the FDA catered to the needs of big business can be found in a crude propaganda piece, "Evaluation of Health Aspects of Sugars Contained in Carbohydrate Sweeteners", recently circulated by the sugar industry, and prepared by the Division of Nutrition and Toxicology, Center for Food Safety and Applied Nutrition, Food and Drug Administration. This report, which strives to exonerate sugar from any connection with obesity, diabetes, hypertension, tooth decay, etc., uses pseudo-scientific language and tables, but is conspicuously short on references. One imagines that the authors of the report were motivated by something other than scientific ideals.

One more example of the FDA's tainted past: For more than a decade, the FDA has refused to recognize the fact that poppers are drugs, and to regulate them as such, claiming that poppers are "room odorizers", since they are labelled as such. The FDA has traditionally been concerned with labelling, and would certainly take action if snake oil were labelled as an "AIDS remedy", or if cocaine were labelled as a "nasal decongestant". Why should they accept the cynically ridiculous claim that poppers are "room odorizers"?[15]

---

[15]John Lauritsen and Hank Wilson, DEATH RUSH: Poppers & AIDS, Pagan Press 1986.

TABLE 5

MORTALITY COMPARISONS
(Four Studies Of AIDS/ARC Patients Treated With AZT)

	Double-Blind Placebo-Controlled Trial	Extended Open-Label Trial	Phase I Trial	Open Market Trial
Bases: Total Patients Participating In Each Trial	(145)	(227)	(33)	(2552)
Deaths During Trial	<1%	10%**	12%**	6%**

* Significantly higher than the Double-Blind, Placebo-Controlled Study at the 99% Confidence Level or more.

** Significantly higher than the Double-Blind, Placebo-Controlled Study at the 95% Confidence Level.

I am also distrustful of the mortality data because of the fact that problems with "drug accountability" were among those found at the delinquent medical center. Suppose that some of the placebo deaths were really AZT patients who had been posthumously reassigned? There are a number of ways that this could have been done. As a check it would be desirable to have some way of verifying that the placebo patients who died really had been placebo patients. Unfortunately, the causes of death were listed in perfunctory and even incorrect ways ("AIDS", "pneumonia [unspecified]", "suspected TB or CMV" or "suspected MAI or CMV"). Since death was not an endpoint of the study, many of the causes of death were not verified.

No autopsies were performed. These might have yielded useful information, and would have verified whether or not there were traces of AZT or other drugs in the bodies of the "placebo" patients.

Project Inform requested copies of the medical records of the patients who died. It would have been possible to determine from these, with considerable accuracy, whether or not the patient had been treated with AZT. The FDA refused to release the medical records, claiming that they were "confidential". It is hard to see why the records would have been "confidential" if the FDA had whited out the names of the patients. And the FDA knows well enough how to white out things. What exactly is the FDA afraid of?

The inadequate descriptions of causes of death, the lack of verification of death causes, the lack of autopsies, the refusal to release medical records — these things are even more suspicious in light of the stringent procedures that the FDA laid down for trials of other drugs. In a recent trial of Ribavirin, autopsies were obligatory, and a Death Report form of more than 30 items had to be filled out for each patient who died.

Efficacy

The mortality data are even more suspect in light of the fact that the "double-blind, placebo-controlled" trial failed to demonstrate that AZT had any benefits, relative to the placebo group. Slight increases in the T-4 cell counts in the AZT group did not persist over time. There is no known mechanism by which AZT could produce benefits sufficient to account for the dramatic differences in mortality.

AZT was found to have "no significant antiviral activity against a variety of other human and animal viruses, including herpes simplex virus type 1, cytomegalovirus, adenovirus type 5, measles virus, rhinovirus 13, bovine rotavirus, and yellow fever virus. It has been shown to inhibit the replication of Epstein Barr virus (EBV)...though the clinical significance of this finding is unknown."[16]

Although AZT (Retrovir) is officially defined as a drug for "symptomatic HIV infection", it was no more effective against HIV than the placebo was. Several measures of viral activity were used, and "no statistically significant changes in the percent of positive cultures or time to detection of virus in culture were observed."[17]

After reviewing the failure of AZT to prove efficacious in any known way, an FDA analyst concluded that AZT treatment is likely to be worse than the disease in the long run:

> Of particular concern is the possibility that the hematologic toxicity of the drug when administered over a prolonged period of time may eventually debilitate patients to such an extent that they may become less able to resist opportunistic infections and other complications of

[16]Cooper, "Medical Officer Review...", p. 128.

[17]Ibid. p. 34.

HIV-disease [sic] than if they had been left untreated.[18]

Toxicity

In summarizing adverse reactions to the drug, the FDA medical officer states, "The majority of patients who were randomized to receive AZT in this trial experienced significant toxicity."[19]   This is, if anything, an understatement, especially considering that many AZT patients were treated with the drug for only a few weeks. If all AZT patients had been treated for 24 weeks, as originally planned, the percentages experiencing various toxicities would undoubtedly have been even higher.

Macrocytosis (enlarged red blood cells, associated with pernicious anemia) occurred in 69% of the AZT patients, but in none of the placebo patients. This measure, which clearly distinguished AZT from placebo patients in over two-thirds of the cases, played a major role in the unblinding of the study among the doctors.

In addition to the "double-blind, placebo-controlled" trial, many experiments were performed, which further demonstrated the high toxicity of the drug. The results of the Cell Transformation Assay suggested:

AZT may be a potential carcinogen. It appears to be at least as active as the positive control material, methylcholanthrene.[20]

---

[18]Ibid. p. 131.

[19]Ibid. p. 39.

[20]Harvey I. Chernov, Ph.D.; "Review & Evaluation Of Pharmacology & Toxicology Data", p. 4.

TABLE 6

BLOOD TOXICITY
(Double-Blind, Placebo-Controlled Study)

	Treatment	
	AZT	Placebo
Base: Total Who Began Trial	(145)	(137)

EXPERIENCED DURING TRIAL:

ANEMIA		
Moderate (Hb < 7.5)	25%*	4%
Severe (Hb < 3.5)	13%*	2%
Hemoglobin decreases > 2g.	38%*	2%
TRANSFUSIONS		
Had at least one transfusion	31%*	10%
Had multiple transfusions	21%*	4%
MARROW SUPPRESSION		
Grade 3 marrow suppression (Hb < 7.5g./deciliter, neutrophile < 750, or white cells <1500)	45%*	12%
MACROCYTOSIS (ASSOCIATED WITH PERNICIOUS ANEMIA)		
Mean corpuscular volume <100μm³	69%*	-
Mean corpuscular volume <110μm³	41%*	-
LEUKOPENIA (white blood count <1500)	27%*	7%
NEUTROPENIA (neutrophile counts <750)	16%*	2%

* Significantly higher than Placebo at the 99% Confidence Level or more.

The FDA analyst who reviewed the pharmacology data, Harvey I. Chernov, succinctly summarized the effect of AZT on the blood:

Thus, although the dose varied, anemia was noted in all species (including man) in which the drug has been tested.[21]

Chernov concluded his review of the pharmacology data by recommending that AZT should not be approved:

In conclusion, the full preclinical toxicological profile if far from complete with 6-month data available, but not yet submitted, one-year studies to begin shortly, etc. The available data are insufficient to support NDA approval.[22]

Ethical issues

There is no doubt that AZT is a highly toxic drug, that it will be harmful to patients, many of whom are already severely debilitated. On the other hand, there is no scientifically credible evidence that AZT has benefits of any kind. The "double-blind, placebo-controlled" trial of AZT is unworthy of credence. Assurances from representatives of the pharmaceutical industry or the Public Health Service, that AZT represents the "best hope", are also unworthy of credence.

I submit that it is malpractice for physicians to prescribe AZT, a poison which can only harm the patient.

I submit that it was unethical for AZT to be approved on the basis of research which was, to put it as generously as possible, invalid.

---

[21] Ibid. p. 7.

[22] Ibid. p. 8

The nation's blood supply belongs to all of us. If AZT continues to be administered to thousands of patients — apparently there are almost 10,000 patients on AZT, at last count — this will mean an intolerable drain on the blood supply, with many AZT patients requiring transfusions as often as every other week. It is one thing when someone becomes seriously ill or has an accident or major operation. Such a person has every right to receive blood. But AZT is now creating entirely another category of patient — those whose bone marrow becomes irreversibly damaged, whose continued existence is forever dependent upon the blood of others. A category of iatrogenic vampires. And this is gratuitous, the result of a drug that should never have been administered in the first place. In this sense AZT harms all of us, not just the patients who are being poisoned by it.

#

III. The Epidemiology of Fear

Psychological warfare is being waged against gay men in the United States. For the past month or so the media have been disseminating hostile propaganda, with the message that we will all die, that we must die. These death threats do not issue from the usual bigots -- not from Roman Catholic agitators, or menopausal beauty queens, or fundamentalist TV hustlers, or quack psychiatrists, or Hasidic zealots. We are not being drummed to death by voodoo witch doctors, or anathematized by prurient priests. We are being cursed in the name of science, and the imprecations directed against us have the imprimatur of the Public Health Service (PHS). The prognosis of doom is emanating from that peculiar form of medical survey research known as "epidemiology".

HIV Antibodies = Death?

Michael Specter, writing in the Washington Post, was one of the first to propound the death message:

The AIDS virus will almost certainly kill everyone it infects unless effective drugs are developed to treat it, federal researchers have predicted for the first time....

After studying a group of gay men from San Francisco for the past decade, however, researchers have produced a statistical model that predicts 99 percent of those infected will eventually develop acquired immune deficiency syndrome 'if they do not die from other causes.'

Because no one has ever been cured of AIDS, a 99 percent AIDS rate means that virtually all would die unless a treatment is developed.[1]

---

[1] Michael Specter, "AIDS Virus Likely Fatal To All Infected", The Washington Post, 3 June 1988.

These grim statements are allegedly based on epidemiological research conducted in San Francisco, as discussed in a report that appears in the 3 June 1988 issue of Science, "A Model-Based Estimate of the Mean Incubation Period for AIDS in Homosexual Men".[2] The authors are Kung-Jong Lui, a mathematician with the Centers for Disease Control (CDC); William W. Darrow, of the CDC's AIDS program; and George W. Rutherford, III, of the AIDS Office in the San Francisco Department of Public Health.

The headline on the second page of Specter's article is even more emphatic, "AIDS Infection Proving Fatal in All Cases". After inaccurately describing the San Francisco study, and repeating the latest doomsday estimates from the PHS (300,000 AIDS cases in the U.S. by the end of 1992), Specter lays out the ramifications of the "finding" that everyone with HIV antibodies will develop AIDS:

Public health service officials...hope the new study will encourage those at highest risk to be tested so that they will seek medical attention if needed....

Many physicians are prescribing AZT for their patients who are infected but have not developed AIDS, although the drug has not yet been proven effective for those patients. Public health officials say that this study is likely to encourage other doctors to prescribe it to patients infected with HIV.

Now, let's step back for a moment and observe what's happening here. First, a number of crucial

---

[2]Kung-Jong Lui, William W. Darrow, and George W. Rutherford, III; "A Model-Based Estimate of the Mean Incubation Period for AIDS in Homosexual Men"; Science, 3 June 1988.

semantic distinctions are being obliterated. "AIDS", a condition or disease that is said to be invariably fatal, is now being conflated with "HIV infection", i.e., having antibodies to a retrovirus that has not yet been shown to be harmful.

(Readers of the Native are aware that Peter Duesberg, a molecular biologist at Berkeley, has provided a powerful, and so far unanswered, critique of the hypothesis that HIV is the cause of AIDS.[3])

The concept of AIDS is expanding to encompass not only AIDS-Related Complex (ARC), but also so-called "HIV infection", and even membership in a "high risk group". To be a gay man is becoming more and more equivalent to being a person with AIDS (PWA).

Second, AZT is being promoted as the appropriate treatment for "HIV infection". Persons who test positive for HIV antibodies will now find themselves between the Scylla of AIDS and the Charybdis of AZT poisoning, with the long-term prognosis of the latter being worse than that of the former. This amounts to a reinstatement of the ancient Judeo-Christian death penalty for sodomy. Lovers of other men must die.

Specter was not alone in putting forth this interpretation of the San Francisco study. On 3 June 1988, Paul Reger, a science writer for the Associated Press, wrote: "AIDS eventually will kill 99 percent of the people infected with the virus, according to a new study that says it takes an average of 7.8 years for the disease itself to show up."[4] And a New York

---

[3] For Duesberg's ideas, see: Peter H. Duesberg, "Human Immunodeficiency Virus and Acquired Immunodeficiency syndrome: Correlation but not Causation", Proceedings of the National Academy of Sciences, February 1989.

[4] Paul Reger, "AIDS Prognosis", Associated Press dispatch, 3 June 1988.

Times article by Bruce Lambert, "New York Called Unprepared on AIDS " (14 July 1988)[5], contained a header, "Almost all carriers of the virus are expected to become ill", and quoted Dr. James O. Mason, director of the CDC, as saying, "We have to assume that everyone infected will ultimately become symptomatic."
New York City Health Commissioner, Dr. Stephen C. Joseph, was quoted as saying:
> I don't know anybody in the field who does not agree that eventually the overwhelming percentage of infected people will have serious if not severe symptomology, in the high 80's, 90's -- as close to universal as you get in medicine.[6]

Before analyzing the San Francisco study, which does not support the statements made by Specter, Reger, Lambert, Mason, and Joseph, a basic point needs to be emphasized. Although there is undeniably a correlation between HIV antibodies and the development of AIDS, the correlation is far from perfect, and it is only a hypothesis that the relationship is causal. Duesberg has persuasively argued that, even in patients who are dying from AIDS, HIV remains biochemically inactive, or latent; and that a virus, like anything else, has to do something to get something done. It has yet to be proven, in even a single case, that HIV has played a role in causing AIDS.

The San Francisco Study
The Science article, "A Model-Based Estimate of the Mean Incubation Period for AIDS in Homosexual Men", has the typical shortcomings of reports written by public health officials. In particular, the report con-

---

[5]Bruce Lambert, "New York Called Unprepared on AIDS", New York Times, 14 July 1988.

[6]Ibid.

tains an inadequate description of methodology, which does not even appear in one place; part of the methodology appears on the first page, and then more methodology appears, incongruously, on the second page. So far as I can tell, this is what was done:

A number of epidemiological studies have utilized a cohort of 6709 homosexual and bisexual men who enrolled at San Francisco City Clinic between 1978 and 1980, in order to participate in various studies of hepatitis B. Investigators Lui, Darrow and Rutherford obtained a subsample of 84 of these men, for whom the approximate date of seroconversion could be estimated -- that is to say, men who had a positive HIV-1 antibody test within 12 months of a negative antibody test. The authors offer the following description: "The 84 men include 83 men who were selected at random or returned for hepatitis B vaccine follow-up, could be located and gave written consent for their stored sera to be tested for HIV-1 antibody, and one man who died from AIDS in 1982."

In the time period involved, from 1978 to the present, 21 of the men (25% of the total) developed AIDS. On the average, for these 21 men, the time between seroconversion and a diagnosis of AIDS (allegedly the "incubation period") was 4.8 years.

Using these data, Lui developed an arcane mathematical model, whose projections were intended to estimate two things: 1) the proportion of the total sample of "infected" men who would eventually develop AIDS, and 2) the "mean incubation period" for those who would develop AIDS. He estimated the latter at 7.8 years. With regard to the former, the following conclusion was reached:

From the Report in Science:
Let p be the proportion of infected individuals who will eventually develop AIDS.... The maximum likelihood estimate

of p is 0.99 with a 90% confidence interval
(0.38, 1.00)....

Confronted with this statement, Specter, who is
obviously unfamiliar with statistical language, simply
latched on to the "maximum likelihood estimate" of
99%, and ignored what followed. And yet the statement, "with a 90% confidence interval (0.38, 1.00)" is
crucial. Translated into plain English, the above
statement reads as follows:

> **Translation:**
> Let "p" be the proportion of individuals
> with HIV antibodies, who will eventually
> develop AIDS.... With about 90% certainty,
> p lies somewhere between 38% and 100%.

Note the difference. With only a 90% confidence
interval, the estimate of "p" has a 62 percentage point
spread, all the way from 38% to 100%. Statistically,
this means that the estimate is wildly unstable. In
fact, if someone asked me to analyze data with a
confidence interval anywhere near this large, I'd simply
tell him to go away, and to come back when he had
data worth looking at. Normally in research one
prefers at least a 95% confidence level, in which case,
according to Lui, "p" would be somewhere between 27%
and 100%! At any rate, these statistics are a far cry
from Michael Specter's statement, "The AIDS virus will
almost certainly kill everyone it infects."
    To make sure that I had interpreted the key
statement correctly, I called both Kung-Jong Lui and
William Darrow, and to my near amazement, they both
agreed with me on almost everything. Lui said that
my rewording of the conclusion regarding "p" was correct, and that the statements made in the press had
been inaccurate and misleading. He said that Specter's
statements, which I read to him, were wrong, and that
if Specter had called him, he would have told him so.

Darrow also agreed that media coverage of their article had been far from satisfactory, and that existing data were not adequate to estimate, with any degree of precision, the proportion of all people with HIV antibodies who would eventually develop AIDS.

A Representative Sample?

Even the grossly unstable estimate of "p" (38% to 100%, with 90% certainty) applies only to the sample studied: 84 homosexual/bisexual men, non-randomly selected from the San Francisco City Clinic Study. It would be wrong to assume that this sample was at all representative of the total universe of people with HIV antibodies. This is one of the most basic questions in survey research: How representative is a sample of a particular universe or population? To what extent is one justified in projecting findings from the sample to the target universe?

Michael Specter, in his article of 3 June 1988 says that "The researchers randomly selected 84 of the men for follow-up studies...." This is simply not true. (In research sampling, "random selection" has a precise meaning: namely, that every individual in the population being sampled has an equal and a known probability of being selected.) In fact, the investigators randomly selected 515 HIV-1 seropositive men from the total cohort of 6709, but were only able to determine the year of seroconversion for 84 (of whom one had been dead for 6 years). They settled for what they could get. Therefore, the 84 men may not even be representative of all seropositive men in the total cohort.

Normally reports on survey research contain a description of the sample. A reader wants to know the characteristics of the people studied, so he can have some idea how typical they are of the total population the sample is intended to represent. There is no such description in the Science report. However, William Darrow was also the principal author of another epidemiological report utilizing the San Francisco City Clinic cohort.[7] This report does describe some characteristics of the City Clinic cohort, who were seronegative when first tested (1978-1980). Darrow told me he saw no reason to assume the characteristics of this sample would differ greatly from those of the 84 men in the other study.

These 359 men were, putting it euphemistically, "living in the fast lane". They were indeed "burning the candle at both ends". With regard to recreational drug use, 84% were cocaine users, 64% used amphetamines, 51% used quaaludes, 41% used barbiturates, 20% used needle drugs, and 13% shared needles. The investigators asked about poppers ineptly, but it appears that the great majority of these men were into poppers as well. In the area of sex, 95% practised receptive anal intercourse with steady or nonsteady partners, 57% averaged more than four different sexual partners per month, 44% practised insertive or receptive fisting with nonsteady partners, and 18% shared douching equipment. In terms of medical history, 74% had been treated for gonorrhea, 73% had had hepatitis, 57% had experienced bleeding with intercourse, 30% had been treated for amebiasis, and 28% had been treated for syphilis.

I would like to make two points, as nonjudgmentally as possible. First, if the 84 men studied by Lui, Darrow, and Rutherford were at all similar to the 359 men in the AJPH study, then they can hardly be representative of the total universe of 1.5 to 3 million individuals in the U.S. estimated by the CDC to have HIV antibodies. Second, it would be surprising if people who lived like this did not become seriously

---

[7]William W. Darrow, Dean F. Echenberg, et al.; "Risk Factors for Human Immunodeficiency Virus (HIV) Infections in Homosexual Men"; American Journal of Public Health, April 1987.

sick; a lifestyle of heavy drug use, multiple venereal diseases with frequent antibiotic treatment, and unhealthy and dangerous sexual practices, may be quite sufficient to cause a condition of immune deficiency, with or without HIV or any other specific infectious agent.

Refutation: New York Blood Center Data

A basic principle of analysis is that data must make sense. This may seem too obvious to mention, but novice analysts often are slaves to the numbers they see in front of them, and will concoct bizarre explanations rather than come to grips with contradictions in the data. In actual practice, when data don't make sense, it is almost always because they are wrong. There are many ways that errors can occur in survey research -- from outright cheating, to errors in coding or study design or mathematics or sampling, to a finger slip on the part of the keyboard operator entering computer tabulation specifications. It is the task of a good analyst to spot and track down such errors.

In the case of epidemiological research, the data ought to make sense in the context of what is known about AIDS. If the findings from the Lui, Darrow and Rutherford study are to have predictive value beyond the 84 men studied, then they should bear comparison with other studies of seropositive individuals.

A study conducted at the New York Blood Center flatly contradicts the findings of the Lui study. According to a New York Times article by Lawrence K. Altman, "AIDS Mystery: Why Do Some Infected Men Stay Healthy?" (June 30, 1987)[8]:

> In New York, at least 13 men who volunteered in 1978 for the hepatitis B vaccine trial were already

---

[8]Lawrence K. Altman, "AIDS Mystery: Why Do Some Infected Men Stay Healthy?", New York Times, 30 June 1987.

infected with the AIDS virus [sic] and have lived for nine years without developing AIDS, according to Dr. Cladd E. Stevens, the head epidemiologist at the New York Blood Center.

An astonishing point is that the immune systems for all 13 of these men look 'perfectly normal,' Dr. Stevens said in an interview....

More astonishing, Dr. Stevens said, for unknown reasons only one of the 87 people in the New York Blood Center study who were found to have become infected with the AIDS virus [sic] since 1981 has developed AIDS.

So then, in New York only one out of 100 "infected" individuals (1%) developed AIDS, whereas in San Francisco 21 out of 84 (25%) developed AIDS. If HIV is the sole cause of AIDS, it is not possible for both sets of data to be correct, notwithstanding the possibility that the time periods may not be quite the same, or that the characteristics of the two samples may be different. The possibility that the difference (25% vs. 1%) could be due to chance is less than one in a million. If, on the other hand, AIDS is caused by toxins (like recreational drugs) and other lifestyle factors, then both sets of data might be correct -- it would mean that the San Francisco subjects pursued an AIDS lifestyle (or "deathstyle"), and the New York subjects didn't, and that in either case, HIV had little or nothing to do with the outcome.

Conclusions

Existing data do not support claims that all, or most, or even many individuals with HIV antibodies will develop AIDS. As usual, government "epidemiology" falls far short of the standards of professional survey research. However, in the present comedy of errors, the main culprits appear to be the media. Reporters like Michael Specter, lacking the necessary training, are not up to the task of interpreting AIDS epidemiology.

It is still nothing more than a shaky hypothesis that HIV has anything at all to do with causing AIDS. In a couple of weeks, an issue of Science is scheduled to run a forum or debate on the HIV hypothesis, with Peter Duesberg arguing that HIV does not cause AIDS; and Robert Gallo, William Blattner and H.M. Temin arguing that it does. It will be the first time that Gallo & Co. have been willing to defend their hypothesis in a civilized manner and in an appropriate publication, complete with references. I suspect that many readers of this debate will be shocked when they realize how skimpy, indeed pathetic, the arguments on behalf of the HIV hypothesis are. And of course, if HIV is not the cause of AIDS, what exactly is the point of attempting to estimate the proportion of HIV-infected individuals who will develop AIDS? Why not estimate the proportion of Judy Garland listeners who will develop AIDS? It might be higher.

It is serious when death threats are directed against us. I sometimes think that too much attention and sympathy have been given to gay men who are sick and dying, and not enough to those of us who have healthy minds and healthy bodies. We are also targets of psychological warfare. We also are increasingly being portrayed as sources of pollution, as threats to the "innocent" heterosexual population.

Our survival depends on not accepting the role of victim. If people direct death wishes at us, we should direct death wishes right back at them. No one should be allowed to attack us with impunity. At the same time we need to retain a sense of cool: an appropriate balance of self-preservation, anger, and a sense of humor. Aside from the fact that our lives are at stake, current events really are pretty absurd, aren't they?

#

IV. On The AZT Front: Part One

It's now more than a year since the New York Native published my analysis of the Phase II AZT trials, which were the basis of the drug's hasty approval by the Food and Drug Administration (FDA). In that article ("AZT on Trial") I demonstrated that the FDA-conducted trials of AZT were not merely sloppy, but fraudulent. In the meantime, a lot of water has gone under the bridge. On the one hand, Burroughs-Wellcome, the manufacturer of AZT (now known as Retrovir) has launched a world-wide propaganda juggernaut, with great success: the majority of physicians treating AIDS patients now prescribe and even proselytize for AZT, and thousands of gay men (including those with AIDS, with ARC, and merely with antibodies to HIV) are being dosed with the drug. On the other hand, there is now a groundswell of opposition to AZT, based on shared experience concerning the drug's side effects. This column will review some recent developments.

Surviving and Thriving With AIDS

The People with AIDS Coalition has just published Surviving and Thriving With AIDS: Collected Wisdom, Volume Two.[1] This large book, written entirely by PWAs and their friends and family, is worth more than dozens of the "medically correct" AIDS books that have flooded the market. As did the first volume, it contains a wealth of practical information. Many photographs and personal accounts vividly document the experience of being a PWA.

---

[1]Michael Callen, ed.; Surviving and Thriving With AIDS: Collected Wisdom, Volume Two. $20 plus $1.75 postage from: People with AIDS Coalition, 31 West 26th Street, New York, NY 10010.

A variety of viewpoints and approaches are expressed on treatments, though on the whole most contributors favor non-toxic therapies. In an article, "Surviving and Thriving with AIDS", Michael Callen, who conducted a study of long-term survivors (who "had survived full-blown CDC-defined AIDS for three or more years"), observes:

Despite intense pressure among physicians to take AZT—the only federally approved treatment for AIDS—only one of the gay long-term survivors was on AZT at the time of these interviews. [The single exception subsequently discontinued taking AZT.]

This is to be expected. The AZT philosophy, based on the assumption that "AIDS is a terminal disease", can offer no more than the forlorn hope of "extending life" for a few months (and there is no factual basis for even this modest claim). Long-term survivors, on the other hand, are convinced that they can and will get better. They are endeavoring to strengthen their bodies through a healthy lifestyle: exercise, good nutrition, rest and stress reduction, and avoidance of harmful substances (including cigarettes, alcohol, poppers, and all other "recreational drugs"). Toxic chemotherapy—like AZT—is incompatible with recovery.

Barry Gingell, a PWA who is also an M.D., writes:

The magic drug Retrovir [AZT] which has been foisted on the public as a triumph against AIDS is actually turning out to be a cumulative poison. While it may prolong life in the short term [not true - JL] AZT creates its own set of serious hematologic problems, which may in fact contribute to the disease rather than moderate it.

One of the book's highlights is "The Pros and Cons of Taking AZT: A Round Table Discussion: June 21, 1988", in which a group of PWAs discuss their experiences with AZT. Some of the main points emerging from the discussion are the tremendous pressure from doctors and peers to take AZT; the hopes, delusions, and subsequent disappointments involving the drug; and the very real and horrible side effects. I cannot imagine that any PWA who reads this 18-page article thoughtfully would have the slightest inclination ever to try AZT.

A common theme is that the discussion participants feel much better, and sleep better, after they cease taking AZT. For example:

SCOTT: I'm feeling better than I've felt in a long time. And a lot of it I attribute to being off the AZT. It was only within the last week that I've actually started sleeping a five hour period. On AZT, I'd wake up after half an hour and then I couldn't go back to sleep. Then I'd fall asleep for an hour and then I'd be up again for another couple of hours.... That might have been the cause of a lot of the fatigue during the day. I can't pinpoint the cause of the sleep problems exactly, but I do attribute them to the AZT.

Another PWA comments:

JEREMY: Since I stopped taking AZT, my stomach hasn't felt bloated; my appetite has been much better and that is good for my general feeling of wellness. Recently I've been sleeping more than usual, which may be because my body needs it and I'm just catching up.... When I was taking AZT around the clock, I wasn't getting as much sleep. Or when I did sleep, they were lots of little naps instead of one uninterrupted daily sleep.[2]

---

[2]Jeremy was subsequently persuaded by his doctor to go on a quarter dose of AZT. He died several months later.

Another participant, Frederick Glenn, states that in general his health has been good since his diagnosis of PCP:

FRED: The only hospitalizations which I have actually incurred were due to the AZT. Twice I ended up in emergency rooms in a state of severe confusion, temperatures, nausea, headaches, which after extensive testing they had to attribute to the AZT. I was transfused three times.

In addition to incapacitating anxiety, Frederick Glenn suffered anemia so severe that he was incapable of dressing himself. Finally one doctor realized that Glenn was having a toxic reaction to AZT, which was causing the anxiety attacks, and recommended he discontinue the drug. The result of going off AZT was an immediate and dramatic improvement:

FRED: I stopped the AZT. And the mental confusion, the headaches, the pains in the neck, the nausea, all disappeared within a 24-hour period. Now, there has to be some correlation there. There has to be. And the minute those symptoms disappeared, my anxiety disappeared with them.

At one point Michael Callen asked the others if they knew anyone who had been on AZT for a year or more, who was doing well, and who experienced no side effects. All of them shook their heads "no". This is significant, because among themselves the discussion participants probably knew thousands of PWAs, including many hundreds who were on AZT.

An exchange between Mike Callen and Kenny Taub offers real insight into the psychology of patients who continue to have faith in AZT, despite the very real suffering they have to undergo, and despite the lack of tangible benefits from the drug:

MIKE: Can you tell us about what opportunistic infections you had during the two and one-half years that you've been on AZT?

KENNY: OK. I've had PCP four times and tuberculosis once. And that's all.

MIKE: What makes you think AZT is doing you any good if you've had pneumocystis four times and tuberculosis while you were on AZT and while you've also had to have 25 transfusions because of AZT-induced anemia? When you say that you think it's doing you good, what do you mean by that?

KENNY: I don't believe that the AZT could stop any opportunistic infection from occurring.... All I can say is, it has been my choice to go on AZT and to stick with it. I've spoken to many researchers nationwide who were pro-AZT in the sense of increasing longevity. And so I made the choice to stick with it and go through the transfusions, even though, yes, they are a pain in the ass.

MIKE: I still don't understand. You have continued to take AZT for a long time because you think it's doing something. What is it that you think it's doing if you've continued to have opportunistic infections and to have serious side effects from AZT? Were you losing a lot of weight, or having fevers, and have those subsided? Has your mental state improved because of AZT or is there some blood test that you feel you've shown a market improvement on that you attribute to AZT? Something has made you stick with AZT through a lot of transfusions and a lot of opportunistic infections. What is that something?

KENNY: That's a good question. Probably the only answer I can give is that I'm psychologically addicted. There's also an ego thing about it. I want to make the Guiness Book of World Records as the longest AZT freak, or something. [Laughs] And I just...I don't know.

Kenny Taub died on 15 December 1988. He had suffered still more attacks of PCP and tuberculosis, as well as collapsed lungs.

A Panel on AZT at Columbia University

On 19 November 1988, a conference was held at Columbia University, "AIDS: Improving the Odds-1988". On the whole it was a flop. Attendance was far below what was anticipated. The auditorium was barbarously overheated. Little was said that was either new or useful, and much was said that was untrue. Open discussion was not permitted. The many slides that were shown by various speakers were projected on the back wall of the stage in such a way that they could not be seen -- the bottom half of each slide was blocked by the table and panel participants on stage. (Curiously, nobody complained, and perhaps it is just as well.)

The least uninteresting panel was on "Azidothymidine -- safety, efficacy, and use in asymptomatic HIV infection [sic]", moderated by Laura Pinsky, one of the organizers of the conference. The first speaker was Craig Metroka, M.D., Ph.D., who gave a presentation that was almost inhuman in its glibness. Metroka rattled off "complications" associated with AZT, as though these were nothing more than the little words on a bottle of over-the-counter pain killer. The "complications", Metroka assured us, were "completely reversible once AZT is stopped". [I'm not so sure that AZT-induced death is "completely reversible", but then why quibble?] Metroka described the "benefits" of AZT, using as his source the notorious Fischl article, which disingenuously reported on the fraudulent, FDA-conducted Phase II trials of AZT.[3]

---

[3] Margaret A. Fischl; "The Efficacy of Azidothymidine (AZT) in the Treatment of Patients with AIDS and AIDS-Related Complex", and Douglas D. Richman; "The Toxicity of Azidothymidine (AZT) in the Treatment of Patients with AIDS and AIDS-Related Complex"; New England Journal of Medicine; 23 July 1987.

The second speaker was Martin Delaney, Co-Director of Project Inform. His talk represented a sharp about-face. A year and a half ago Delaney was in the Ribavirin camp, and was an important opponent of AZT. It was Project Inform, together with ACT UP, that obtained the FDA documents, under the Freedom of Information Act, which were the basis of my exposé of the AZT trials, as well as the basis of exposés by NBC news and by Joseph Sonnabend, M.D. A year ago this summer, Delaney described the AZT trials in scathingly critical terms.

Delaney has changed his tune, and is now on the Burroughs-Wellcome team. His talk was a hard-sell pitch for AZT. "AZT is not the enemy", pleaded Delaney, "let's not get into a shouting match [?]". He urged the audience not to "argue all day about flaws [only flaws?] in the [AZT trials] study", since it was "necessary to look at all studies of AZT".

Delaney downplayed the toxicity of AZT by claiming that toxicity data "in the most part were coming from very sick patients". A lot of the problems with AZT, he argued, came from giving it to "the wrong people at the wrong time"; the side effects were "far less significant when used in healthier people".

Toxicity out of the way, Delaney began to wax enthusiastic. There were hundreds of patients, he contended, who had been using AZT successfully for one year, two years, and longer. The value of AZT lay in administering it in "early stages of infection" in order to "halt the progression of HIV". Delaney then related an anecdotal case, and advocated using AZT in half doses and in combination with such drugs as dextran sulfate and acyclovir.

Ending on a maudlin note, Delaney lamented, "A lot of people are being discouraged from ever trying AZT." "Give them a chance to use it", he pleaded, "Let's not close the door on this drug until we find something to replace it with!".

The next speaker was Joseph Sonnabend, M.D., M.R.C.P., who has privately published his own critique of the AZT trials.[4]   Sonnabend began by saying that the toxicities of AZT should not lightly be dismissed. The harmful effects of the drug are real, and they are serious.   Technically, AZT is a poison; it is cytotoxic [i.e., it kills cells].   The drug cannot distinguish between infected and healthy cells; it kills both.   Never before has a drug as toxic as AZT been prescribed for long-term use.   The long-term effects of AZT, the cumulative toxicities, are unknown.   Sonnabend emphasized the ethical responsibilities of the physician, to be sure that there was a sound scientific basis for the benefits of the drug, considering that its toxicities were firmly established.

Sonnabend then described some of the shortcomings of the AZT trials, in particular the fact that the study became unblinded early on [i.e., both doctors and patients knew whether AZT or a placebo was being administered].   The basic design of the study was thus violated.   Not only did the unblinding have a powerful psychological effect on the patients, but it may have led to unequal and biased patient management from the attending physicians.

After Sonnabend finished his presentation, he was attacked by Martin Delaney, who maintained that he had seen a lot of patients go back to work, that not all studies of AZT were meaningless, and that at least a dozen other studies had produced similar results.

Michael Lange, M.D., spoke next, concentrating on a single point: whether an antiviral effect against HIV has been demonstrated scientifically for AZT.   Lange acknowledged that some scientists were convinced that

---

[4] Joseph A. Sonnabend, "Review of AZT Multicenter Trial Data Obtained Under the Freedom of Information Act by Project Inform and ACT-UP", AIDS Forum, January 1988.

HIV is not the cause of AIDS. Nevertheless, it is claimed that AZT works by preventing HIV from replicating, and this claim ought to be examined. Lange then proceeded to review all of the data, both published and unpublished, that bore on the question. He concluded that evidence for an antiviral effect of AZT on HIV was completely lacking. Two years ago, in early 1986, claims were being made that AZT inhibited HIV, on the basis of the P-24 antigen test. However, at the FDA hearings held in early 1988, there was no talk of the P-24 antigen test; it had not panned out. Lange criticized the way AZT had been promoted by the "Medical Industrial Complex", stressing that we do not know what the long-term effects of the drug are.

The next speaker was Ron Grossman, M.D., who immediately launched into a personal attack on Joseph Sonnabend: "With all due respect, Joe, no drug is not poison — you know that well — there are far more poisonous drugs than AZT!" [Grossman's statement is pure demagoguery. What other drugs are as toxic as AZT? And have they been prescribed for long-term use by healthy people?]

Doing his best to pooh pooh the toxicities of AZT, Grossman asserted that every other drug in medicine also had toxic effects. He went so far as to claim, "We know more about the toxic effects of this drug than about any other drug studied." [This is a blatant falsehood. Since no more than a handful of people have taken AZT for more than two and a half years, the cumulative toxicities of the drug are totally unknown.] Grossman went on to describe the AZT trials in glowing terms, arguing that the speedy approval of AZT showed, "There aren't just bad guys in Washington." Grossman ridiculed the notion that co-factors (like poppers or other drugs) played a role in causing AIDS: "The only co-factor is time. We know that." He concluded by saying that AZT slowed the progression of HIV, the drug bought "quality time", and "AZT offers hope".

Next, Michael Callen, of the PWA Coalition, described the "overwhelming peer pressure to take AZT".
In response to Grossman's claim that AZT "offers
hope", Callen suggested it would be better to offer
hope through substances that didn't have the serious
toxicity of AZT. "It is not rational", said Callen, "to
say that everyone with AIDS ought to try AZT. The
arguments against AZT are very well developed, and
very rational, and what we ought to do is make certain
that everyone has access to the arguments on both
sides of the issue." "There are those of us who made
a rational choice not to try AZT", he stated, "and we
need to support those who have decided not to take
AZT, just as we have supported those who are taking
AZT."

In the discussion period, both Sonnabend and Lange
commented that poor quality science had been used on
behalf of AZT, and asked Martin Delaney to state
specifically what studies he had in mind. At this point
Delaney became truculent: "I don't have a list of
studies in my briefcase, but there were page after page
in the [Stockholm] abstracts supporting positive results
from studies of AZT. And if necessary, I'll meet with
you privately [?!] to show you some of these studies."
Delaney's diatribe continued: "Let's not pretend that
there's even a significant minority opinion out there
that suggests AZT is not an antiviral. I can't find
anyone outside this table to suggest that that's the
case.... The AZT argument is becoming a magnet for
anti-establishment feelings. That's not OK when lives
are at stake."

Sonnabend, maintaining his dignity, replied that he
had looked at the Stockholm abstracts, and that the
quality of evidence was soft. The abstracts involved
uncontrolled observations of small numbers of patients;
for scientific debate, they were little better than
anecdotal evidence. Grossman then snapped at Sonnabend, "That's poppycock! Everyone at the table
except you knows that's rubbish!"

Laura Pinsky, who as moderator ought to have attempted to keep Delaney and Grossman to some measure of civility, instead joined the pack and told the audience that Sonnabend and Lange were "very much a minority". Her comment was gratuitous and unfair, and caused one gentleman in the audience to proclaim, "That doesn't mean they're wrong!" At this point I raised my hand and attempted to speak, Pinsky screamed that there would be "no discussion from the floor". The panel was over.

I then went up on stage, and asked Pinsky when there would be an open discussion, as I wanted to correct a number of untrue things that had been said during the panel. Pinsky told me, not very courteously, that there would be no open discussion, and that if I had a question I should write it on a piece of paper like everyone else. I then approached Grossman, and asked him if he had read my article on the AZT trials. Grossman's response was to snarl something inarticulately and to turn his back on me. When I returned to my seat, a security guard approached me, and said he had been asked to "escort" me from the building. I and the people with me were amazed, to say the least, but it was time for the lunch break, so I let myself be escorted out.

Later in the day, during an afternoon panel, I left the auditorium to go to the men's room, and was intercepted by the same guard, who said he had been asked to see that I didn't enter the auditorium. I told him that everything was all right, and not to worry, and went back in, half expecting him to follow. He didn't.

After the conference was over, I asked Pinsky why a guard had tried to keep me out of the auditorium. She denied knowing anything about it, and said I should point out the guard to her. Perhaps Pinsky was telling the truth, but she is no friend of free speech. Last summer Pinsky, and her colleague Paul Douglas, went around Fire Island, as official representatives of

Gay Men's Health Crisis (GMHC), telling gay men that they should get themselves tested for HIV antibodies, and if "positive", should consider going on AZT. At one of these talks, a Fire Island resident took issue with some of Pinsky's and Douglas's statements concerning the causal role of HIV and the benefits of AZT. Pinsky's response was to ask the audience to agree with her that he should not be allowed to speak. On this occasion she played the wrong card, for on Fire Island it was she who was the outsider, and the audience emphatically indicated they wanted to hear what their friend had to say. Pinsky and Douglas did not attempt to answer his arguments.

The Columbia conference was an unpleasant experience for me. I don't like having security guards called on me because someone is afraid of my presence: that I might say something out of place or write an article for the New York Native. I don't like showcase conferences devoted to creating delusions so fragile that they would be shattered by free and open discussion. This is totalitarianism.

#

V. On The AZT Front: Part Two

In my previous article, "On The AZT Front: Part One", I concluded there is no scientifically credible evidence that AZT has benefits of any kind. Nevertheless, the popular media and medical journals are filled with statements to the effect that AZT has been shown to "extend life". This claim appears to be based on three bodies of "research":

First, there are the Phase II ("Double-Blind, Placebo-Controlled") AZT trials, conducted by the Food and Drug Administration (FDA)[1]. In "AZT on Trial", I demonstrated that the FDA-conducted trials of AZT were not merely sloppy, but fraudulent, and that government approval of AZT was therefore improper and illegal.

Second, there are a number of abstracts which were presented at the AIDS conference held in Stockholm last summer. These consist of unpublished data derived from uncontrolled observations of small numbers of patients; for scientific debate, such reports, in the context of a conference where 3200 abstracts were presented, are no better than anecdotal evidence.

Third, there is a major study of AZT, "Survival Experience Among Patients With AIDS Receiving Zidovudine [AZT]", which has just appeared in the 25 November 1988 issue of the Journal of the American Medical

---

[1]Margaret A. Fischl; "The Efficacy of Azidothymidine (AZT) in the Treatment of Patients with AIDS and AIDS-Related Complex", and Douglas D. Richman; "The Toxicity of Azidothymidine (AZT) in the Treatment of Patients with AIDS and AIDS-Related Complex"; New England Journal of Medicine; 23 July 1987.

Association (JAMA).[2] The purpose of this article is to show that this is very bad research, on which no credence of any kind should be placed.

The AZT Philosophy

The toxicities of AZT are firmly established. The drug is cytotoxic (i.e., it kills healthy cells); it destroys bone marrow; it causes severe anemia, headaches, nausea, and muscular atrophy; it damages the kidneys, liver, and nerves; and it inhibits DNA synthesis. The consequences of AZT toxicity should not be taken lightly. When DNA synthesis is blocked, new cells are not formed, cells do not develop -- the life process in effect comes to a halt. Joseph Sonnabend, a prominent New York City AIDS researcher and physician, expressed it succinctly: "AZT is incompatible with life."

The question then arises: How can physicians justify prescribing this drug, whose benefits are so dubious and whose side effects are so terrible? Physicians are supposed to honor the Oath of Hippocrates, the cardinal principle of which is to act for the good of the patient, doing nothing that is harmful. But AZT is harmful. In the words of molecular biologist Peter Duesberg, "AZT is pure poison."

I suggest that the answer to this paradox can be found in the common belief that AIDS is "invariably fatal", that people with AIDS (PWAs) have only a few months to live. The JAMA article expresses this cornerstone of the AZT philosophy: "AIDS is a terminal

---

[2] Terri Creagh-Kirk et al., "Survival Experience Among Patients With AIDS Receiving Zidovudine [AZT]: Follow-up of Patients in a Compassionate Plea Program", Journal of the American Medical Association, 25 November 1988.

disease".[3]   Physicians who accept this premise may be
able to prescribe AZT in good conscience: since PWAs
are considered to be facing imminent death, the cumulative toxicities of AZT can be ignored, and AZT
therapy can be rationalized as offering the hope of
"extending life" for a few months (though there is no
factual basis for even this modest claim).

There are several objections to the AZT philosophy.
Most important is the fact that AIDS is not invariably
fatal.   There are PWAs who have survived for many
years, who are leading full and productive lives, and
who appear by all rational criteria to be recovering.
And why not?   What other disease is "invariably fatal"?
I imagine that future medical historians, looking back
on the present, will regard many or even most of the
AIDS fatalities as iatrogenic -- caused by medical
treatments rather than by AIDS itself (whatever exactly "AIDS" is).   It is noteworthy that long-term survivors, almost without exception, have avoided toxic
chemotherapy (like AZT) and have opted for strengthening their bodies through a healthy lifestyle: exercise,
good nutrition, rest and stress reduction, and avoidance
of harmful substances (including cigarettes, alcohol,
poppers, and all other "recreational drugs").   PWAs
deserve a chance to recover.   With AZT there is no
chance.

AZT is now being tested on healthy people who
merely have antibodies to HIV, which according to
Duesberg is a typically harmless retrovirus.   Members
of the AIDS establishment, like William Haseltine, have
advocated giving AZT to seronegative members of "high
risk groups" (meaning us, gay men).   To do so would
be tantamount to genocide.

The poisoning of sick and healthy people alike with
AZT is a cruel hoax, inasmuch as there is still no hard
scientific evidence to support claims of AZT benefits,

---

[3]Ibid. p. 3014.

least of all in the latest "research" emanating from Burroughs-Wellcome.

The JAMA Article

When the Phase II AZT trials were abruptly terminated in September 1986, it was anticipated that government procedures would require about six months before AZT could be marketed for prescription use. An interim measure was established, whereby AIDS patients who had previously experienced an episode of Pneumocystis carinii pneumonia (PCP) could receive AZT prior to marketing of the drug. This was done on a "compassionate plea" basis under a "Treatment Investigational New Drug (IND)" exemption, the rationale being that these patients were "at substantial risk of early death" and AZT would benefit them, presumably by preventing further attacks of PCP. The JAMA article, "Survival Experience Among Patients With AIDS Receiving Zidovudine [AZT]", reports on 4805 patients who received AZT under this IND program.

Collaborating in the study were the National Institute for Allergy and Infectious Diseases, the National Cancer Institute (NCI), the Food and Drug Administration (FDA), Burroughs Wellcome (the manufacturer of AZT), and Biospherics Inc. (apparently a private research company located in Beltsville, Maryland). It was hoped that the program would provide "an opportunity to gather data regarding longer-term experience with zidovudine" in a population that was larger and more varied than that in the Phase II trials.

Children were totally, and women almost entirely, excluded from the study. The average age of the 4805 subjects was 37 years; 97% of them were male, 87% were "homosexual or bisexual", and 79% were "white, not Hispanic". It is stated that "Many patients reported more than one AIDS risk behavior" -- in other words, many of the gay men were also intravenous drug users -- and yet this overlap has been suppressed in the JAMA article's Table 1.[4] (See Exhibit 1.)

Table 2.—Description of Enrolled Population Undergoing Zidovudine Treatment

Characteristic	No. (%) of Patients
Risk category	
Homosexual/bisexual	4168 (86.7)
Intravenous drug abuser	287 (6.0)
Hemophiliac	65 (1.4)
Heterosexual	184 (3.8)
Transfusion recipient	66 (1.4)
Unknown	35 (0.7)
Gender	
M	4658 (96.9)
F	147 (3.1)
Race	
White, not Hispanic	3798 (79.0)
Black, not Hispanic	520 (10.9)
Hispanic	424 (8.8)
Pacific Islander and American Eskimo	21 (0.4)
American Indian	3 (0.1)
Other	39 (0.8)

EXHIBIT 1. This table is reproduced exactly from the JAMA article, p. 3011. It is clear that most (87%) of the victims of "zidovudine treatment" are gay men. Notice that the overlap group, gay men who are also IV drug users, has been suppressed; these patients are counted only as "homosexual/bisexual", but not as "IV drug abuser". The total number of patients (4805) is not shown, suggesting that the authors and/or editors of JAMA are ignorant of a basic statistical convention.

---

[4]Ibid. p. 3013.

Each patient was initially dosed with 200 mg of AZT every four hours around the clock. However, provision was made to lower the dosage or to discontinue dosage temporarily, in the case of "adverse effects". Approximately 1500 physicians cooperated in the study by enrolling or following up patients. These doctors were told, when they agreed to participate, that they would be expected to supply information on their patients on a regular basis. Before September 15, 1986 patient information came in automatically, since doctors needed to provide it in order to obtain further supplies of AZT for their patients. After September 16, 1986 data collection became more haphazard, though the investigators tried to continue obtaining data through telephone contact and mailed questionnaires.

Missing: 1120 Patients

In the interests of fairness, I called Burroughs Wellcome, to hear their explanations for what appear to be incompetence, dishonesty, and fraud connected with this research. I spoke briefly with Terri Creagh-Kirk, MS, the principal author of the JAMA article, and at greater length with David W. Barry, MD, also an author of the article and Burroughs Wellcome Vice President in charge of research. I'll say this much for Burroughs Wellcome: at least their people are courteous and willing to talk -- in sharp contrast to the NCI and the CDC, where military security measures prevent unauthorized reporters (whether from the Native or the BBC) from talking to the so-called "scientists". I found the explanations of the Burroughs Wellcome researchers to be completely unacceptable, but at least they have some respect for dialogue. In an atmosphere of intensifying censorship and totalitarianism, this is appreciated.

For some reason the Burroughs Wellcome researchers set their sights on reporting 44 week (or 10 month) survival for the AZT recipients. Unfortunately, by this time they had completely lost control of the study. It had bombed. Incredible as it sounds, nearly one out of four subjects (23%) had been lost. The researchers did not know whether 1120 patients were even dead or alive -- and if alive, whether or not they were still taking AZT. (See Table A. Please note that in this article the lettered tables are my own, whereas the "Exhibit" tables are reproduced from the JAMA article, with my own comments at the bottom.)

TABLE A

SURVIVAL STATUS AFTER 44 WEEKS OF AZT TREATMENT

	Total Patients
Base:	4805 = 100%
Survival Status After 44 Weeks...	
Reported alive	2838 = 59%
Reported dead	847 = 18%
Unknown (i.e., lost)	1120 = 23%

If one looks only at the 1043 patients who were enrolled in the first four weeks of the IND program, the record of the Burroughs Wellcome researchers is even more appalling. No fewer than 734 (70%) of these patients had been "lost". (See Table B.)

TABLE B

SURVIVAL STATUS AFTER 44 WEEKS OF AZT TREATMENT
(Among Patients Enrolled in the First 4 Weeks)

	Total Patients Enrolled In First 4 Weeks
Base:	1043 = 100%
Survival Status After 44 Weeks...	
Reported alive	309 = 30%
Unknown (either dead or lost)	734 = 70%

Terri Creagh-Kirk explained that they had tried hard to find out what had happened to the 1120 patients who were lost (letters, telephone calls, etc.). I am not impressed. Professional researchers are expected to anticipate problems before they occur. To lose track of nearly one-quarter of an entire study group is colossal incompetence, for which there can be no excuses. If a professional researcher ever found himself responsible for such a disaster, he would probably be contemplating two courses of action: exile or suicide. But not the intrepid Burroughs Wellcome researchers -- they decided to resort to some statistical hocus-pocus, in order to pretend that the 1120 patients hadn't really been lost after all.

A Guess Is A Guess Is A Guess

Of the 4805 patients, 2838 (59%) were reported as being alive after 44 weeks -- if we assume that all of the "lost" patients had died, then 59% would represent the lowest possible survival estimate. On the other hand, 3958 patients (82%) were not reported to have died after 44 weeks -- if we assume that all of these patients were indeed alive, then 82% would represent the highest possible survival estimate. The true percent surviving presumably lies somewhere in between 59% and 82%. The Burroughs Wellcome researchers used some kind of statistical projection technique in order to estimate -- or guess, as it were -- what the true percent surviving would be if all the data were in and the 1120 patients had not been lost.

This is an abuse of statistics. Projection techniques are not a form of magic. The fact is that the Burroughs Wellcome researchers lost control of their study. They failed. And there is no form of statistics that can remedy this, any more than it can put spilt milk back in the bottle or put Humpty Dumpty back together again. Terri Creagh-Kirk said that the Kaplan-Meier Product Limit method had been used to estimate the percent surviving after 44 weeks. However, the Kaplan-Meier Product Limit method is not mentioned in the JAMA article, which refers to a "LIFETEST procedure" and to "standard survival techniques", whatever those might be.

After all the the talk about the Kaplan-Meier Product Limit method and/or the LIFETEST procedure, it is something of a letdown to find that the authors may have obtained their 73% estimate by a simpler method. They state that if all the "lost" patients were still alive (and on AZT), "the survival at 44 weeks could be estimated to be as high as 82%". On the other hand, if all of the "lost" patients had "died 15 days after the last report was received [a peculiar assumption, but let it pass]", the "survival could be estimated to be as low as 64%". At this point they add together the two percents (82% + 64%) and divide by two, thus obtaining -- Eureka! -- an average of 73%. Having performed elementary school arithmetic they write: "The true survival falls somewhere between these two points, presumably most closely reflected by the overall point estimate of 73%."[5]

Whatever projection techniques were used, the authors of the report reach the conclusion: "Overall survival at 44 weeks after having started therapy was 73% ($\pm$2.1%) (Fig. 12)".[6] At this point I wish to emphasize two things. First, the use of the word, "was". The authors did not write, "was estimated to be", which would have been honest; they wrote, "was", which is a lie. Unless specified otherwise, a percent is always assumed to be an actual percent. Second, the confidence interval of $\pm$2.1% is impossibly low, considering that it must reflect not only the error inherent in a projection trying to compensate for the loss of 23% of the total sample, but must reflect sampling variation as well. (See Exhibit 2.)

On the first page of the article it is stated: "A detailed description of data management and tracking procedures is beyond the scope of this article and will be published elsewhere." When I talked to Creagh-Kirk she said she had just begun to write this "description". I look forward eagerly to reading it, but in the meantime we already know enough to reject and repudiate what the Burroughs Wellcome researchers have done. They have deliberately and fraudulently presented an estimate as though it were an actual percent (derived by dividing an actual number by an actual total). That these people intended to deceive is evident from the statement in the abstract at the beginning of the JAMA article: "Overall survival at 44 weeks after initiation of therapy was 73% ($\pm$2.1%)."[7]   Nowhere in

---

[5] Ibid. p. 3013.

[6] Ibid. p. 3012.

[7] Ibid. p. 3009.

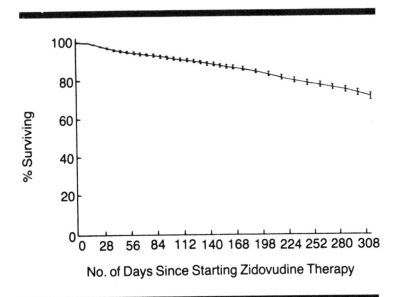

Fig 1.—Overall survival experience of patients with acquired immunodeficiency syndrome undergoing zidovudine therapy (with confidence limits).

EXHIBIT 2. The above chart is reproduced exactly as it appeared in the JAMA article, p. 3014. Note that there is plenty of white space between the bottom two bars, which could have been used to explain that the chart is based on statistical estimates rather than actual percents. Note further that the annotation on the y axis reads "% Surviving", which is misleading and fraudulent. There is plenty of room to say "Estimated % Surviving" or "Est. % Surviving".

the abstract is there even a hint that the 73% figure is merely an estimate.   It goes without saying that an abstract should accurately summarize the main article, since many people never read beyond the abstract.

David Barry claimed that Burroughs Wellcome had no control over these matters, that they were dictated by the editorial policy of JAMA.   This is nonsense.   It is not for the JAMA editors or anyone else to decide that a guess is just as good as an actual statistic. Nor is it for them to decide whether or not tables and charts need to have sufficient annotation that they will be meaningful and truthful.

Unexplained Deaths

Since the focus of the study was on survival versus death, it is obviously important to know the causes of death for the 847 patients who are known to have died.   The inadequacy of the information obtained reveals once again the incompetence of the researchers.   At the very beginning of the study, the physicians ought to have been told that they would be expected to provide complete and accurate information on their patients.   Therefore it is disconcerting to learn that the single most frequent cause of death was described as "unspecified" (16.4%).   (See Exhibit 3.) And if we add together "unspecified" (16.4%) with "AIDS, not classified" (11.2%), we find that fully 27.6% of the deaths were described in unacceptably vague and meaningless terms.   Further, we observe that there are no fewer than three "causes" related to pneumonia, which might or might not be the same thing: "pneumocystis carinii pneumonia" (13.8%), "respiratory arrest" (7.2%), and "pneumonia unspecified" (6.0%); together these three add up to 27%.[8]   A professional analyst would have "netted" together the three forms of pneumonia — showing the "net" total on the table, with the

---

[8]Ibid. p. 3012.

Table 4.—Most Frequently Reported Primary
Causes of Death Among Patients With AIDS
Undergoing Zidovudine Therapy*

Cause of Death	Frequency	% of Deaths
Unspecified	139	16.4
Pneumocystis carinii pneumonia	117	13.8
AIDS, not classified	95	11.2
Mycobacterial disease	75	8.9
Respiratory arrest	61	7.2
Neoplasm	56	6.6
Pneumonia, unspecified	51	6.0
AIDS with infection, no neoplasm	39	4.6
Septicemia	37	4.4
Encephalopathy, acute	26	3.1
Cachexia	25	3.0
Cardiac arrest	24	2.8
Lymphoma	24	2.8
Cytomegalovirus	23	2.7
AIDS with infection, neoplasm	22	2.6
Disorder of central nervous system	20	2.4
Dementia	19	2.2
Inanition	19	2.2
Blood loss	11	1.3
Cryptococcal meningitis	11	1.3
Meningitis	11	1.3
Toxoplasmosis	11	1.3
Seizures	10	1.2
AIDS with neoplasm, no infection	9	1.1

*Multiple causes of death were reported for many
patients. All attributed causes of death have been
included. AIDS indicates acquired immunodeficiency
syndrome .

EXHIBIT 3.   Note that 27.6% of the deaths are either
"unspecified" or "AIDS, not classified".   No fewer than
three "causes" are related to pneumonia, which might
or might not be the same thing (Pneumocystis carinii
pneumonia, respiratory arrest, and pneumonia unspecified); together these add up to 27%.   The authors fail
to show the total number of deaths (N = 847) on which
the frequencies in the first column are percentaged.

three specific forms of pneumonia underneath the net. David Barry did not know what "netting" meant, although it is an elementary statistical procedure, and one which is essential to produce meaningful tables.

Faulty Comparisons

Even if one accepted the 73% survival at 44 weeks after initiation of AZT therapy, one would still have to ask whether this survival rate is really very good. The authors of this study believe that it is, and state: "The survival estimate for this treated cohort is significantly above that described in previously reported natural history cohorts." They then proceed to make a number of specious comparisons to:

- An old (1981-1985) New York City cohort where the median cumulative survival was estimated to be 10.5 months.

- A fragment of the CDC's AIDS statistics, focussing only on cases diagnosed in the first six months of 1986.

- A study of one year [not 44-week] survival for hemophiliacs [a congenitally sickly population] with AIDS.

- A "prospective" study of a San Francisco cohort showing only 50% surviving beyond 11.2 months [not 44 weeks or 10 months]. This so-called "prospective" study is merely an abstract presented at a June 1987 AIDS conference.

None of these "natural history" studies is at all comparable to the IND study reported on in the JAMA article. Besides which, there are numerous and major problems involved in attempting to make survival comparisons: Do AIDS patients who take AZT have the same characteristics as those who do not take

AZT? Probably not. Do PWAs on AZT receive the same patient management as PWAs who are not on AZT? Probably not. Are PWAs living longer now than they were a few years ago? They probably are (and this could be because patient management is better, or because PWAs being diagnosed now are not as sick as those being diagnosed several years ago). In addition there is the fact that about 50% of PWAs cannot tolerate AZT and have to be taken off the drug. What this means is that the stronger patients (taking AZT because they can tolerate it) are compared with the weaker patients (who cannot tolerate AZT). Obviously this is a strong bias in favor of AZT.

Speaking with a forked tongue the authors of the JAMA article say:

> The use of historical controls is intended simply to provide a reference point, and no attempt is made to make statistical comparisons between the natural history cohort and this population of zido-vudine-treated patients.[9]

This caveat is definitely called for. Any such comparison would be invalid. Nevertheless, the JAMA article had no sooner appeared in print than the Burroughs Wellcome researchers rushed to the media to claim that AZT had extended the lives of the patients in the IND study. An Associated Press dispatch of November 25, 1988 reported that:

> Nearly 5,000 people who took the AIDS-fighting drug once known as AZT survived at a much greater rate than those without it, say researchers for the medicine's maker.

According to the AP story Terri Creagh-Kirk said that "records of people who were diagnosed with AIDS before zidovudine became available show only 50%

---

[9]Ibid. p. 3015.

survived past 11 months". This is a reference to the "prospective" San Francisco cohort study, a completely improper comparison. The disparity between the caveat in the JAMA article, and the subsequent statements made by the authors of the JAMA article to the media, suggests that these people intend to deceive.

Summing Up

It is disgraceful that the editors of JAMA allowed this garbage to be published. It is disgraceful that they permitted a dubious estimate to be palmed off as an actual survival statistic, and that they permitted false and misleading comparisons to be made. In no way does this study show that AZT "extends life" or is even slightly beneficial. The study demonstrates only how farcical are the peer-review standards of even the leading medical journals.

#

VI. AZT And Cancer

It is urgently necessary to review the toxicity of AZT in light of recent marketing developments. Prior to last August, AZT therapy was officially indicated only for "AIDS" or "ARC" patients who either had "a history of cytologically confirmed Pneumocystis carinii pneumonia (PCP) or an absolute CD4 (T4 helper/inducer) lymphocyte count of less than 200/mm^3 in the peripheral blood before therapy is begun." (Physician's Desk Reference) This changed dramatically in August, when a series of press releases were issued by the National Institute of Allergy and Infectious Diseases (NIAID) and other branches of the Public Health Service (PHS), claiming that AZT was beneficial for "HIV-infected" persons with "mild symptoms of immune system damage" and also for "HIV-infected persons who have not yet developed symptoms."

The old rationale for prescribing AZT was that people with AIDS (PWAs) were suffering from a disease that was invariably fatal, that such persons had only a few months to live, and that AZT might extend their lives for a few more months. The idea was that in a desperate situation, drastic measures were called for. I have repeatedly argued that this viewpoint is wrong -- that "AIDS" is not invariably fatal; that some PWAs have survived for many years and appear to be recovering; and that the only chance for recovery lies in strengthening the body, rather than injuring it through toxic chemotherapy like AZT.

Now a completely different game plan is in operation. With well-orchestrated propaganda emanating from NIAID, Gay Men's Health Crisis (GMHC), Project Inform, and various and sundry other "AIDS" groups, clinical researchers, and other confederates of Burroughs Wellcome (the manufacturer of AZT), physicians are now being urged to prescribe AZT for perfectly healthy people. The targeted individuals--

estimated to be several hundreds of thousands in the United States alone -- merely have antibodies to HIV-1, a retrovirus that has not yet been proven to be harmful, let alone the cause of the devastating AID Syndrome. Healthy people, who ought to look forward to living for several more decades, are now being conned into taking the most toxic substance ever prescribed for long-term use. Since gay men are the primary targets of AZT marketing, since AZT therapy would probably cause even an athlete in his prime to die within a few years, and since the alleged "benefits" of AZT rest upon fraud, it is not unreasonable to use the word "genocide" to describe what is happening.

The Great AZT Scam: Results Without Data

In my articles in the Native I have analyzed the studies that allegedly demonstrate AZT's effectiveness, and have concluded that there is no scientifically credible evidence that AZT has benefits of any kind. Documents which the Food and Drug Administration (FDA) was forced to release under the Freedom of Information Act revealed that the Phase II ("double-blind, placebo-controlled") AZT trials were worthless. The researchers covered up the fact that the study had become unblinded (thus violating the basic test design). Protocol violations were overlooked. Worst of all, the researchers deliberately used data that they knew were false. These fraudulent trials were the basis of government approval of the drug.[1]

Another study often cited as proof of AZT's benefits concerns patients who received AZT after the

---

[1] Native Issue 235.   Another highly critical review of the Phase II trials was written by Joseph A. Sonnabend, "Review of AZT Multicenter Trial Data Obtained Under the Freedom of Information Act by Project Inform and ACT-UP", AIDS Forum, January 1988.

Phase II trials were prematurely terminated.[2]   I have
written an extensive analysis of this study, which is a
rotten mixture of incompetence and dishonesty.[3]
Through colossal incompetence the researchers lost
track of 1120 patients, not knowing if they were even
alive or dead.   They then used statistical projection
methods to guess what results they would have obtained if they had not lost the 1120 patients, presented
their guesses as actual survival statistics, and made a
number of grossly invalid comparisons in order to claim
that AZT had extended lives.   This "research" is a
blatant exercise in disinformation, proving nothing
except how farcical are the "peer review" standards of
medical journals.

As appalling as these two studies were, they at
least presented data, however dubious.   The two studies that received so much fanfare last August didn't
even go that far.   The general public, physicians,
PWAs, and health care workers were expected to
accept "findings" which consisted of generalizations
that were not even backed up by numbers.   Normally a
press release on a study is issued a few days before
the publication of a report in a peer-reviewed medical
journal.   This is ethically obligatory, because physicians with the responsibility of prescribing a drug--
especially one as toxic as AZT -- are entitled to have
recourse to hard data, a proper description of methodology, and an intelligent analysis of the findings.

On 17 August 1989 the U.S. Department of Health

---

[2]Terri Creagh-Kirk et al., "Survival Experience
Among Patients With AIDS Receiving Zidovudine [AZT]:
Follow-up of Patients in a Compassionate Plea Pro-
gram", Journal of the American Medical Association, 25
November 1988.

[3]Native Issue 300.

and Human Services (HHS) issued a press release, which began:

> A multicenter AIDS drug trial with more than 3,200 volunteers has shown that zidovudine (AZT) delays progression of disease in certain HIV-infected persons who have not yet developed symptoms.

The alleged findings of the study (known as ACTG Protocol 019) were described in a vague paragraph, which did not give a single hard statistic:

> The Board found that, in those participants with fewer than 500 T4 cells who received zidovudine [AZT], the rate of progression to AIDS or severe ARC was roughly half that for participants with fewer than 500 T4 cells who received placebo. Progression to symptoms was about the same in patients receiving either 500 mg per day or 1,500 mg per day of the drug. Toxicities were minimal in both treatment groups. More importantly, with the exception of nausea that occurred in about 3 percent of the volunteers, virtually no differences in side effects were observed in persons receiving the lower dose and persons receiving placebo. (From press release, U.S. Department of Health and Human Services, 17 August 1989)

Then on 24 August 1989 NIAID issued its own press release, "Results of Controlled Clinical Trials of Zidovudine in Early HIV Infection". This two-pager covered both Protocol 019 (healthy persons) and Protocol 016 (persons with "mild symptoms"), and gave even less information than the HHS statement had. It made the highly implausible assertion that "zidovudine toxicity experienced by the persons studied in Protocol 019 was minimal."

I spent several days calling NIAID and various other PHS branches in an attempt to obtain some hard information about Protocol 019. They sent me a three-page "Backgrounder" entitled, "ACTG 019 - Questions and Answers". This Q & A described the "results" of the study in one paragraph.

What were the actual results? Zidovudine [AZT] delayed the onset of advanced ARC or AIDS for individuals who entered the study with less than 500 T4 cell counts. As of August 10, 1989, 38 individuals randomized to placebo had developed endpoints (33 of which were AIDS). Only 17 individuals randomized to 100 mg zidovudine five times daily had developed endpoints (11 of which were AIDS), and 19 individuals receiving 300 mg five times daily developed endpoints (14 of which were AIDS). The substantial difference in outcome between treatment groups was observed for those entering the study with a T4 cell count less than 500. However, for individuals entering with T4 cell counts between 500 and 800, fewer endpoints occurred, and no definite statement regarding differences in event rates can be made at this time. (From "Backgrounder: ACTG 019 - Questions and Answers", National Institute of Allergy and Infectious Diseases, 17 August 1989)

As the reader can see, this statement is gibberish, it gives no real data, and it is in contradiction with the earlier HHS press release.

When I talked to the NIAID press officer who was supposed to be most knowledgeable about Protocol 019, and asked him some specific questions (which he was unable to answer), he told me frankly that I had all of the information he himself had -- that there was nothing he could tell me I didn't already know.

Based on my knowledge of Protocol 019, equal perhaps to that of anyone in the country, I constructed Table 1, which shows the findings in the simplest and most straightforward way possible. This table should be studied carefully by anyone who is considering the use of AZT for an "asymptomatic HIV-infected person". Table 1 contains all of the data we have about Protocol 019.

TABLE 1

"Results" From NIAID-Conducted Protocol 019:
Placebo-Controlled Trial In Asymptomatic HIV-Infected Persons

	Total Sample*		Treatment			
			AZT		Placebo	
Bases:	(?)		(?)		(?)	
	#	%	#	%	#	%
Progressed to "AIDS" or "Advanced ARC"***	?	?	?	?	?	?
Duration of Treatment:						
Range (months)	(?)		(?)		(?)	
Mean (months)	(?)		(?)		(?)	
Median (months)	(?)		(?)		(?)	

*According to NIAID, "more than 3200 asymptomatic HIV-infected volunteers" were enrolled "approximately two years ago". However, all studies have drop-outs. NIAID does not state how many volunteers were still participating when the study was terminated.

**Also sometimes referred to as "severe ARC" (undefined).

Drug Regulation American Style

The ordinary mind often fails to make the distinction between things as they are and things as they ought to be. For example, if the FDA is to do its job and protect the American public from dangerous drugs, it ought to have a system for keeping track of adverse reactions to a drug after it has been put on the market. Many people therefore assume that there is such a system. There is not. In this regard the United States takes an approach to drug regulation that is different from that of most other industrialized countries.

In the United States, all of the efforts in screening a new drug for adverse side effects are supposed to take place before the drug is approved. Once a drug has been approved -- whether by hook, crook, or the intrinsic merits of the product -- it's clear sailing from then on. In theory, physicians are supposed to report adverse effects to manufacturers, who are supposed to relay the information to the FDA. But in practice, with no incentives for compliance, no punishments for noncompliance, and with no federal data gathering system, the post-marketing surveillance is haphazard at best.

In contrast, Britain has a sophisticated and rigorously enforced system of post-marketing surveillance. The philosophy there is that some adverse effects of a drug only become apparent after a certain period of time -- this is known as chronic toxicity -- and that some adverse effects might be relatively rare, found perhaps in only 1 in 1000, or 1 in 5000 persons. Neither the chronic toxicity nor the rare adverse effects would likely be identified in pre-marketing trials, which typically involve only a few hundred subjects treated for a relatively short time.

Most new drugs take 9 to 10 years to go through the FDA's approval process, which includes initial safety tests in animals and human beings, clinical trials for efficacy and safety, and extensive review and analysis of the data.   AZT, however, was rushed through the approval process faster than any drug in the FDA's history — less than two years.   As a result, the officially recognized toxicities of AZT are far from complete.   Further, the "non-official" toxicities of AZT, well known through the formidable PWA grapevine, are not being systematically recorded.

On top of all these problems, AZT was approved on the basis of research that was not just inadequate, but fraudulent.   It is important to realize that the FDA has been for many decades a notoriously corrupt agency.   Time and again officials in the FDA have colluded with drug manufacturers in order to suppress information about a drug's side effects.   Recently Dr. Sidney M. Wolfe, director of the non-profit Public Citizen Health Research Group (HRG), charged that under Commissioner Frank E. Young, the FDA "is implicitly inviting all of the industries it regulates to join in the lawlessness."[4]   I am preparing a future article that will review some of the well-documented crimes against public health that have been committed through collusion of drug manufacturers, the FDA and other branches of the Public Health Service, clinical researchers, and the American Medical Association.

The Chernov Review of AZT's Pharmacology & Toxicity
Among the documents which the FDA was forced to release under the Freedom of Information ACT was the "Review & Evaluation of Pharmacology & Toxicology Data" for the drug Retrovir (generic name: zidovudine, aka AZT or azidothymidine), written by FDA toxicology

---

[4]Morton Mintz, "Anatomy of a Tragedy", New York Newsday, 3 October 1989.

analyst Harvey I. Chernov, Ph.D., and submitted in its final form on 29 December 1986.[5]

Chernov reviewed several dozen studies that had been completed, including in vitro studies and experiments on rats, mice, rabbits, beagle dogs, and human beings. Many additional studies had not been completed or had been planned but not begun. The single most important finding was that AZT was toxic to the bone marrow, causing anemia. Chernov wrote:

Thus, although the dose varied, anemia was noted in all species (including man) in which the drug has been tested.

Chernov noted that AZT "was found weakly mutagenic in vitro in the mouse lymphoma cell system. Dose-related chromosome damage was observed in an in vitro cytogenetic assay using human lymphocytes."

Evidence from the "Cell Transformation Assay" indicated that AZT was likely to cause cancer. In Chernov's summary:

This BALB/c-3T3 neoplastic transformation assay was performed according to standard operating procedure. Concentrations of AZT as low as 0.1 mcg/ml reduced the number of cells in culture after a 3-day exposure. A statistically significant increase in the number of aberrant 'foci' was noted at a concentration of 0.5 mcg/ml. This behavior is characteristic of tumor cells and suggests that AZT may be a potential carcinogen. It appears to be at least as active as the positive control material, methylcholanthrene [a known and extremely potent carcinogen].

---

[5]Harvey I. Chernov, Ph.D., Review & Evaluation of Pharmacology & Toxicology Data, NDA 19-655, 29 December 1986. (FDA document obtained under the Freedom Of Information Act).

Chernov was concerned that in the rush to approve AZT, the FDA was violating its own guidelines and proceeding on the basis of inadequate information:

> FDA guidelines would have prescribed more extensive preclinical testing than that reported thus far. However, the urgency for developing an anti-AIDS drug has been so great that clinical testing has preceded the usual/customary preclinical testing. For example, while data from a 6-month clinical study are available, results of the supporting 6-month preclinical toxicity studies have not yet been submitted. Also, the applicant has a protocol for a 104-week clinical study, whereas chronic (52-week preclinical toxicity studies are not scheduled to start before January-February of this year.

Taking into account all of the information available to him, Chernov recommended that AZT should not be approved for marketing:

> In conclusion, the full preclinical toxicological profile is far from complete with 6-month data available, but not yet submitted, one-year studies to begin shortly, etc. The available data are insufficient to support FDA approval.

AZT and Cancer

Obviously if AZT is going to be prescribed to healthy (if "HIV-infected") people, with the expectation that they will take the drug for the rest of their lives, it is important and ethically imperative that physicians and patients be fully informed on the issue of carcinogenicity. But Burroughs Wellcome and their accomplices in the FDA have done their best to sweep carcinogenicity under the rug. Back in 1986 Burroughs Wellcome proposed dealing with the results of the Cell Transformation Assay by saying on the Retrovir label, "The significance of these in vitro results is not known."

This proposed labelling was criticized by the FDA toxicology analyst, Harvey Chernov, for being misleading:

> The sentence: "The significance of these in vitro results is not known." is not accurate. A test chemical which induces a positive response in the cell transformation assay is presumed to be a potential carcinogen.[6]

Burroughs Wellcome resolved this problem by simply dropping the offending sentence, with the end result being every bit as obscurantist. In the Retrovir entry in Physicians' Desk Reference, written by Burroughs Wellcome, carcinogenicity is dealt with in the following way:

> Long-term carcinogenicity studies of zidovudine in animals have not been completed. However, in an in vitro mammalian cell transformation assay, zidovudine was positive at concentrations of 0.5 mcg/ml and higher.

Well now, how many physicians would know what these findings meant? Damned few, if any. Chernov said what the findings meant: AZT is presumed to be a carcinogen! But most physicians would assume that AZT was not carcinogenic, for the simple reason that the Physicians' Desk Reference entry hadn't said it was.

In toxicology a basic distinction is made between acute toxicity and chronic toxicity. Acute toxicity refers to those adverse effects that are manifest within a relatively short period of time (if not necessarily immediately). Chronic toxicity refers to adverse effects that only become apparent over time. It is a truism of toxicology that chronic toxicity cannot be predicted from acute toxicity.

---

[6]Harvey Chernov, op. cit..

There are several kinds of chronic toxicity. In one kind, a single exposure to the substance can result in illness many years later -- this appears to be the case with Agent Orange (dioxin).   Another kind of chronic toxicity involves an accumulation of the substance within the body, after which symptoms occur.   Still another kind of chronic toxicity involves the accumulation of injury:

Consider the circumstances of a small degree of irreversible injury resulting from each of a series of doses. If the change effected by a single divided dose is truly irreversible, the end result of a series of doses may be essentially identical with the effect of the same total dose given at one time.[7]

It takes time to determine the potential of a substance to cause cancer. This is one reason why Chernov objected to the approval of AZT before the completion of long-term carcinogenicity studies.   In the words of a toxicology expert:

Time as well as dose is a factor in assessing properties of chemical carcinogens as compared to drugs.   It is in this way that carcinogens differ from ordinary toxic agents.   A number of small doses give no overt signal of their presence and in due time can yield tumors within the life-span of a host.   With noncarcinogens such low dosages would be completely innocuous.'[8]

---

[7]Louis J. Casarett, 'Toxicologic Evaluation', a chapter in Toxicology: The Basic Science of Poisons, edited by Louis J. Casarett, Ph.D., and John Doull, M.D., Ph.D., New York, Toronto, and London, 1975.

[8]John H. Weisburger, 'Chemical Carcinogenesis', a chapter in Casarett and Doull, op. cit..

The point regarding "low dosages" is especially relevant in the case of AZT. Many PWAs have been led to believe that if they are on low dosages of AZT, they will evade the terrible toxicities of the drug. Perhaps they will to some extent evade the acute toxicities, but only time will tell what chronic toxicities lie in wait, including cancer.

Samuel Broder of the National Cancer Institute (NCI) is the man who is more responsible than anyone else for the development and promotion of AZT. (For this role, some "AIDS dissidents" have nominated Broder for the annual Dr. Josef Mengele award.) Even Broder now admits that his drug may cause cancer. He is co-author of a recently published article in the New England Journal of Medicine (NEJM), in which it is stated:

> In considering early intervention with zidovudine, it is of particular concern that the drug may be carcinogenic or mutagenic; its long-term effects are unknown.[9]

Having made this admission, the authors engage in some strangely sophistical reasoning: "Zidovudine may be associated with a higher incidence of cancers in patients whose immunosurveillance mechanisms are disturbed, simply because it increases their longevity." Of course, other things being equal, increased longevity increases one's risk for all kinds of things, including perishing in an earthquake, dying of old age, or having dinner with an anti-porn activist. However, Broder & Company are wrong to assert that AZT increases longevity, for "patients whose immunosurveillance

---

[9] Robert Varchoan, Hiroaki Mitsuya, Charles E. Myers, and Samuel Broder, "Clinical Pharmacology of 3'-Azido-2'3'-Dideoxythymidine (Zidovudine) and Related Dideoxynucleosides", New England Journal of Medicine, 14 September 1989.

mechanisms are disturbed". I challenge them, or anyone else, to cite a single, scientifically credible study, that proves this.

Muscular Atrophy and Other Unofficial AZT Side Effects

As mentioned above, there is no official, on-going surveillance of AZT's side effects. Nevertheless, we have a pretty good idea what some of them are from the PWA grapevine. And occasionally some unofficial side effects surface in letters to medical journals or in off-the-cuff comments at AIDS conferences. One such side effect is muscular atrophy coupled with intense muscular pain. Many PWAs have experienced this condition, for example, Peabody in San Francisco:

> After being on a full dose of AZT for about 10 months, I started to go downhill -- more fatigue, headaches, nausea/dizzy feeling, painful intestinal cramping AND loss of mass in my legs. I'm not sure if this loss of mass is muscle or fat. I lost about 8 lbs and was having sciatic like leg pains. I went off the AZT completely and now I feel almost normal. Much more energy, less of the other symptoms. BUT I'm worried about my skinny legs and bony butt. My doctor thinks it's HIV related -- but what do doctors know! I had the leg pain and loss of mass while on the AZT and feel better off the AZT.[10]

Another PWA, Diogenes, wrote:

> I had the same experience on AZT with leg pain and muscle loss. Been off AZT 2 mos. now and pains are almost completely gone -- also muscle

---

[10]Communication from Peabody, Public Forum, AIDS Information Bulletin, San Francisco: (415) 626-1246.

soreness and loss of muscle tone has reversed some-
what.[11]

Instances of severe muscular atrophy and pain
caused by AZT were reported in a letter to the New
England Journal of Medicine. The physicians observed:

All patients had an insidious onset of myalgias,
muscle tenderness, weakness, and severe muscle
atrophy favoring the proximal muscle groups.
Physical examinations revealed varying degrees of
muscle weakness and grossly apparent atrophy.
Weight loss due to muscle loss was uniformly noted;
in one patient, the loss was a striking 18 kg. [40
pounds].

The physicians held AZT responsible for the muscular atrophy and pain:
We did not observe this illness before zidovudine
was available, the disorder was seen in patients
taking the drug for extended periods, and the
syndrome was ameliorated after the drug was
stopped.[12]

A leading British AIDS doctor, Dr. Matthew Helbert,
sent Burroughs Wellcome stock into a temporary
tailspin when be publicly commented on muscular
atrophy and other serious, but not officially acknowledged, side effects of AZT:
Biting hard on the hand that had paid his air
fare, he placed heavy emphasis on new, debilitating

[11]Communication from Diogenes, ibid.

[12]Laura J. Bessen et al., "Severe Polymyositis-
Like Syndrome Associated With Zidovudine Therapy of
AIDS and ARC" (letter), New England Journal of Medi-
cine, 17 March 1988.

and sometimes deadly side-effects of Retrovir on some of his Aids patients.   Some men's muscles had degenerated dramatically after long-term use of the drug.   Others had rapidly developed a serious brain disease, encephalitis, soon after being taken off the drug.   Given the company's duty to keep a new drug under active surveillance, Dr. Helbert asked why the company had not picked up similar cases among the thousands of people treated with Retrovir for a year or more in the United States.[13]

Other well-known, but not officially acknowledged, side effects of AZT include damage to the kidneys, liver, and nerves.   An old friend of mine was one of the earlier patients to be put on AZT.   Everyone thought he was doing well.   For almost a year he was occasionally able to work or go to concerts.   Then one day he went into complete paralysis, and he died two days later.   Now, paralysis is not an officially recognized side effect of AZT; there is no warning about it on the package.   Nevertheless, there is a connection.

Peter Duesberg has referred to AZT as a "poison", and with good reason.   AZT is cytotoxic — it kills cells.   AZT terminates DNA synthesis, the very life process itself, by which new cells are formed and grow.   Therefore, damage to each and every organ of the body is an expected consequence of AZT therapy.

Ethics

I believe that history will severely condemn the ethical shortcomings of such AZT promoters as Samuel Broder, Anthony Fauci, and Margaret Fischl.   In their zeal to expand the market for AZT, they have unconscionably failed to inform the public about the likely long-term consequences of AZT therapy.

---

[13]Duncan Campbell, "The Amazing Aids Scam", The New Statesman, 24 June 1988.

I also believe that history will condemn the physicians, "AIDS groups" and individuals who have been urging healthy ("HIV-infected") gay men to take AZT.

Two years ago I wrote in the Native that "It is malpractice for physicians to prescribe AZT, a poison which can only harm the patient."[14] I reaffirm this judgment. When physicians coax and cajole and bully their "HIV-positive" patients into taking AZT, do they tell them that the long-term effects of AZT are unknown?...that AZT is cytotoxic?...that AZT destroys bone marrow?...that AZT causes muscular atrophy and pain?...that AZT terminates DNA synthesis?...that AZT damages the nerves, kidneys, and liver? Do they tell their patients that AZT will probably cause cancer in the long run? If not, these physicians have failed to inform their patients about the dangers of a drug whose "benefits" have yet to be demonstrated.

And I issue this challenge to the AZT doctors. If you know of a single scientifically credible study-- just one — which proves that AZT is beneficial -- for PWAs, for people with ARC, for healthy ("HIV-infected") people, or for anyone else -- then let me know. I would certainly acknowledge it publicly.

Dr. Joseph Sonnabend, one of the most intelligent and honest AIDS researchers, has said that "AZT is incompatible with life." In a recent conversation Sonnabend said that Fauci, Fischl, and the other AZT advocates have been remiss, and indeed criminally negligent, in not mentioning the likelihood that long-term use of AZT may result in cancer. I believe that ten years from now, looking back over tens of thousands of horrible, AZT-related deaths, no reasonable person will disagree with his verdict.

#

---

[14]Native Issue 235.

VII. Burroughs Wellcome Issues Advisory

AZT causes cancer in animals. This finding was divulged by Burroughs Wellcome, manufacturer of AZT (also known as Retrovir, zidovudine), in an advisory sent on 5 December 1989 to thousands of physicians who treat AIDS patients. Widespread consternation ensued. Confused and contradictory statements were issued to the press by physicians, Public Health Service (PHS) officials, and "AIDS activists".

The study involved 960 male and female rats and mice, which were treated for 19-22 months, equivalent to most of their normal lifespan. High, middle, or low doses of AZT were administered to 720 of the rodents, while the other 240, as controls, received nothing. Cancer occurred only among the female rodents treated with AZT. Seven of the 60 female mice receiving the high dose, two of the 60 female rats receiving the high dose, and one of the 60 female mice receiving the middle dose developed cancer of the vagina. No tumors were found in any of the control rodents. The cause-effect relationship between AZT and the cancers was real and significant; according to the investigators, in a group of this size, in this amount of time, there should have been no cancers of the type observed.

Immediately promoters of AZT rushed in to downplay the significance of the findings. In an Associated Press story, Dr. James Mason, assistant secretary for health of the Department of Health and Human Services said that the results "do not establish that the drug has a carcinogenic effect in humans." Along the same lines, Burroughs Wellcome stated in its letter that "results from rodent carcinogenicity studies are of limited predictive value for humans." These are strange things to say. If rodent carcinogenicity studies have little "predictive value for humans", why do them in the first place? If rodent studies are meaningless, why are they a standard part of the toxicity

screening of new drugs?   Of course, the carcinogenicity of some substances is species-specific.   So what?
There are probably substances that cause cancer in
humans but not in rodents.   The main point of these
findings is that AZT can cause cancer in animals--
therefore it is reasonable and prudent to act on the
assumption that it can cause cancer in humans as well.

Mason further "noted" that the doses given to the
rodents in the study were "much higher than recommended for human use."[1]   This statement is baffling.
Nowhere in the Burroughs Wellcome "Backgrounder" or
letter is it stated that the highest rodent dose of AZT
was higher than the equivalent human dose.   The three
test doses are described simply as high, middle, and
low.   It is unlikely that the highest rodent dose could
have been higher than the equivalent recommended
human dose for one reason: a large proportion of
human beings treated with a full dose of AZT develop
life-threatening anemia and have to be taken off the
drug.   Further, according to a government toxicology
analyst, AZT-related anemia has been found in all
species studied, including rodents, dogs, monkeys, and
human beings.[2]   Therefore, if the rodent dose had
really been extraordinarily high, many of the rodents
would have perished from anemia.   This did not happen.   If anything, the highest rodent dose was probably
well below the equivalent human dose, inasmuch as few
human beings have been able to stay on a full dose of
AZT for more than a few months at a time.   And none
of the rodents were given transfusions.

---

[1]Deborah Mesce, "AZT-Tumors", Associated Press,
5 December 1989.

[2]Harvey I. Chernov, Ph.D., Review & Evaluation
of Pharmacology & Toxicology Data, NDA 19-655, 29
December 1986.   (FDA document obtained under the
Freedom Of Information Act).

Philip J. Hilts wrote in the New York Times: "Doctors who treat many AIDS patients said the findings raised concerns about only one group: pregnant women infected with the AIDS virus."[3]   This is absolutely false, and refuted by (of all people) Burroughs Wellcome public relations spokeswoman Kathy Bartlett, who correctly stated:

Though the rodents developed vaginal tumors, that raises the possibility of a carcinogenic potential in general and should not be interpreted as applying only to the vagina or to women.[4]

In a Reuter dispatch of 5 December, a stock market analyst, Peter Smith, is quoted as saying, "There's no indication at this stage that it affects humans."   This is not true.   As readers of the Native are aware, a standard test for carcinogenicity, the Cell Transformation Assay, was performed over three years ago.   The results were highly positive, indicating that AZT should be "presumed to be a potential carcinogen" -- in humans.   I first cited the Cell Transformation Assay over two years ago[5] and described it in more detail just over a month ago.[6]   And now, in light of the rodent carcinogenicity study, it may be time to look at the findings again.

---

[3] Philip J. Hilts, "AIDS Drug Causes Cancer in Animals", New York Times, 6 December 1989.

[4] Mesce, op. cit.

[5] Native Issue 235.

[6] Native Issue 340.

The Cell Transformation Assay

In 1987 the Food and Drug Administration (FDA) was forced to release, under the Freedom of Information ACT, a large quantity of documents related to the approval of AZT. Among these was the "Review & Evaluation of Pharmacology & Toxicology Data" for the drug Retrovir (generic name: zidovudine, also known as AZT or azidothymidine), written by FDA toxicology analyst Harvey I. Chernov, Ph.D., and submitted in its final form on 29 December 1986.[7]

Chernov reviewed several dozen studies that had been completed, including in vitro studies and experiments on rats, mice, rabbits, beagle dogs, and human beings. Many additional studies had not been completed or had been planned but not begun. The single most important finding was that AZT was toxic to the bone marrow, causing anemia. Chernov wrote:

Thus, although the dose varied, anemia was noted in all species (including man) in which the drug has been tested.

Chernov noted that AZT "was found weakly mutagenic in vitro in the mouse lymphoma cell system. Dose-related chromosome damage was observed in an in vitro cytogenetic assay using human lymphocytes."

Evidence from the "Cell Transformation Assay" indicated that AZT was likely to cause cancer. In Chernov's summary:

This BALB/c-3T3 neoplastic transformation assay was performed according to standard operating procedure. Concentrations of AZT as low as 0.1 mcg/ml reduced the number of cells in culture after a 3-day exposure. A statistically significant increase in the number of aberrant 'foci' was noted at a concentration of 0.5 mcg/ml. This behavior is characteristic of tumor cells and suggests that AZT

---

[7]Harvey Chernov, op. cit.

may be a potential carcinogen. It appears to be at least as active as the positive control material, methylcholanthrene [a known and extremely potent carcinogen].

It should be noted that the Cell Transformation Assay evaluates the effects of substances on human cells. The test is considered to be highly predictive of the potential of a substance to cause cancer in humans. In Chernov's words, "A test chemical which induces a positive response in the cell transformation assay is presumed to be a potential carcinogen."

The results of the Cell Transformation Assay are well known to Burroughs Wellcome, since they are alluded to (if cryptically) on the Retrovir package insert and in the Retrovir entry in the Physicians' Desk Reference. It is regrettable, therefore, that these results were not mentioned in the Burroughs Wellcome advisory letter or in any of the newspaper articles. Physicians who must make an evaluation of the carcinogenic risks of AZT will do so on the basis of incomplete information. They will know about the rodent studies, but not about the equally important Cell Transformation Assay.

Interview With Jerome Horwitz

The impression given by the Burroughs Wellcome letter is that the issue of carcinogenicity was raised for the first time by the rodent studies. This is not true, of course, as the results of the Cell Transformation Assay were known over three years ago. The question then arises whether other information on AZT's carcinogenic potential was available even further back in time.

I telephoned Dr. Jerome Horwitz, the man who invented AZT back in 1964. Horwitz was a little disgruntled, feeling that he had been interviewed enough already, but he agreed to answer some questions. According to Horwitz, AZT was developed in the hopes that it would be effective in treating cancer. AZT was abandoned because it was not effective against cancer; the drug failed to prolong the lives of leukemic animals.   AZT was never tried in human beings, since it completely failed to demonstrate efficacy in the animal studies.

I asked Horwitz what toxicities were observed in the animals, and whether AZT was also rejected because of its extreme toxicity.   He replied that AZT was not rejected because of toxicity, but only because it was not effective against cancer.   I then asked whether cancer had been observed in any of the animals.   At this point Horwitz became quite defensive, and said that he "categorically denied" that cancer had been found.   He asserted that the investigators had been looking only at the prolongation of life in the leukemic animals.   According to him, it was not until the mid-'80s that any animal toxicity studies were done, either by Burroughs Wellcome or by Samuel Broder at the National Cancer Institute.

There is a conflict of testimony here, which I am unable to resolve.   Other reporters have been under the impression that AZT was abandoned in the '60s largely or even primarily because of its toxicity.   For example, Brian Deer wrote in the Sunday Times that AZT had been "abandoned in 1964 as being too poisonous".[8]   Celia Farber, who interviewed Horwitz, wrote in SPIN: "[AZT] had actually been developed a quarter of a century earlier as a cancer chemotherapy, but was shelved and forgotten because it was so toxic, very expensive to produce, and totally ineffective against cancer."[9]   Another colleague, who has requested ano-

---

[8]Brian Deer, "Revealed: Fatal Flaws of Drug That Gave Hope", Sunday Times (London), 16 April 1989.

[9]Celia Farber, "Sins of Omission: The AZT Scandal", SPIN, November 1989.

nymity, has informed me that Horwitz told him in an interview that AZT was abandoned because of its extreme toxicity as well as its ineffectiveness: Not only did AZT not cure cancer, it caused it!

Whatever the truth may be about toxicity studies in the '60s — and I imagine that much information has irretrievably gone down the memory hole -- one fact stands out: AZT was rejected as a cancer drug without ever trying it on humans. Although the impression is sometimes given that AZT is an old cancer drug for which a new use was found, no human being had ever taken AZT until brave volunteers did so in the mid-'80s, as part of the FDA-conducted Phase I (toxicity) trials of AZT.

The Changing Risk-Benefit Ratio

In responding to news about the rodent carcinogenicity studies, a number of AZT apologists sounded a particular theme: The risks of AZT must be weighed against its benefits. For example, James Mason is quoted as saying: "In spite of these new animal findings, patients with the disease appear to be at far greater risk from not receiving zidovudine treatment than from any potential risk of cancer associated with the drug's use."[10]

Patients taking AZT were less glib. Peter Staley, a member of ACT UP, is quoted as saying:

I am taking AZT and I do find this fairly worrisome, but I am more fearful of HIV than I am of cancer. This shifts the equation of benefit and risk, but not enough to tilt it away from using the drug.[11]

---

[10]Mesce, op. cit.

[11]Philip J. Hilts, op. cit.

There is a large and growing body of information on the risks of AZT. In addition to the risk of cancer, AZT is cytotoxic (lethal to body cells); it destroys the bone marrow and causes severe anemia; it damages the kidneys, liver, and nerves; it causes severe muscular pain and atrophy (wasting away). What then are the "benefits" of AZT, that could offset such terrible toxicities?

I have maintained, and continue to maintain, that there is no scientifically credible evidence that AZT has benefits of any kind. This is an open challenge, and I should be grateful if any of the AZT promoters would cite a single study -- just one -- which demonstrates benefits of AZT and deserves to be called "scientifically credible". So far, this challenge has either been evaded completely, or a dozen generally worthless "studies" have been rattled off, with the comment that the evidence is "overwhelming". The latter tack was recently taken in an abusive and ill-informed article in the PWAC Coalition Newsline.[12]

It is legitimate to speak of a "risk-benefit ratio", but first the "benefits" have to be established. It will not do to substitute quantity for quality. A dozen worthless studies prove nothing, even if they all agree with each other. By way of analogy, let's think back on the vast number of flying saucers or "unidentified flying objects" (UFOs) that were observed in the '60s. None of the observations were very well documented, but there were so many of them! How could it be that they were all wrong!?

I take no position on whether or not flying saucers from outer space have visited our planet, either recently or in the past, but merely point out that such visitations remain to be demonstrated. Likewise with the benefits of AZT.

---

[12]Rob Schick, "The Crazy Case Against AZT", PWAC Coalition Newsline, November 1989.

Bad News For Business?

Stock market analysts were puzzled by the fact that the obviously bad news of AZT's carcinogenicity had almost no effect on the share price of Burroughs Wellcome stock. Ian White, pharmaceuticals analyst at U.K. Stockbroker Kleinwort Benson, commented: "I don't understand why the shares have not fallen." White said he would have expected about a 20 pence drop in the share price after the news about the increased "risk factor".[13]   White's lack of concern for the human (as opposed to profit) aspects of AZT therapy is stunningly revealed in his comment:

If cancers do develop in humans, it's probably going to take a while to develop.[14]

The profits from the sale of AZT are enormous. According to the McGraw dispatch:

Retrovir, Wellcome's second-highest-selling product with sales of 134 mln pounds [= $214 million] in the year ended Aug. 26, is widely expected to be one of Wellcome's fastest-growing products in the early 1990s.[15]

Undeterred by the rodent carcinogenicity findings, Burroughs Wellcome expects business to be better than ever in 1990, as the market for AZT expands to include perfectly healthy people who happen to have antibodies to HIV (a retrovirus which, according to renowned molecular biologist Peter Duesberg, is "pro-

---

[13]"Wellcome Says Tests Show AIDS Causes Cancer in Rodents", McGraw-Hill News, 5 December 1989.

[14]"Wellcome Says Retrovir Can Cause Cancer in Rats", Reuter dispatch, 5 December 1989.

[15]McGraw-Hill News, 5 December 1989.

foundly conventional" and therefore presumably harm-less).[16] According to a McGraw-Hill story:

A Wellcome spokesman said the company is reit-erating recent comments by its director of research in the U.S., Dr. David Barry, that Food and Drug Admin. approval for use on asymptomatic HIV-positive patients would be "a matter of months."[17]

Summary

At this point, the best available information indi-cates that AZT will cause cancer in humans. Other toxicities of AZT are severe and well-established. On the other hand, not one single scientifically credible study demonstrates that AZT has benefits of any kind. Therefore, patients with "AIDS" or "ARC", as well as people who are merely "HIV-infected", have nothing to gain and everything to lose by taking AZT.

#

---

[16]Peter H. Duesberg, "Human immunodeficiency virus and acquired immunodeficiency syndrome: Cor-relation but not causation", Proceedings of the Nation-al Academy of Sciences, February 1989.

[17]McGraw-Hill News, 5 December 1989.

VIII. U.S. Cuts AZT Dose In Half

The Food and Drug Administration (FDA) announced on 17 January 1990 that the recommended dose of AZT, the only federally approved drug for "AIDS", would be cut in half. The old dose was 1200 milligrams per day. The new dose will be only half that: 600 milligrams per day after one month at the old dose of 1200 milligrams. The FDA has ordered changes in the labels on AZT (also known as zidovudine or Retrovir) to represent the new recommendation.

For some time prior to the FDA's announcement, doctors who treat "AIDS" patients had been experimenting with lower doses, in an effort to avoid the side effects of the drug. At the old dose of 1200 milligrams, about half of all "AIDS" patients had been unable to tolerate AZT's extreme toxicity, which caused severe anemia, as well as muscular pain and atrophy (wasting away) and damage to the kidneys, liver, and nerves.

Health and Human Services Secretary Louis Sullivan said in a statement that the change "means that fewer patients may have to discontinue AZT therapy because of serious side effects."

The new dose recommendation was based on government press releases from last summer, which allegedly showed that the lower dose was just as effective as the higher, while causing fewer serious side effects. These "preliminary findings" have not yet been written up, let alone published in a reputable scientific journal. Nor have any hard data been released. This practice of "science by press release" was sharply criticized in the pages of the New York Native, as well as in an editorial in the Lancet, one of the world's most prestigious medical journals.

According to those "preliminary findings", nearly half of those receiving the high dose (1200 milligrams) had side effects that were so serious they had to discontinue AZT treatment. At the same time, fully a quarter of those receiving the low dose also had to discontinue treatment, for the same reasons.

It is important to note that the "benefits" of AZT remain unsubstantiated by scientifically credible research. The studies allegedly demonstrating AZT's "benefits" have been very bad. The Phase II trials, which were the basis of FDA approval of AZT, were demonstrably fraudulent, as well as invalid through pervasive sloppiness.

The FDA's action was hailed by "AIDS activists" as being "good news", which in a way it was. As with any poison, the less the better, and lowering the dose of AZT means less immediate injury to the unfortunate patients taking the drug. On the other hand, the bad news is that the lower dose will enable much larger numbers of people to take AZT, thereby exposing themselves to the chronic (long-term) toxicities of the drug. According to the best information we have, which includes rodent carcinogenicity studies and in vitro studies involving human cells, the long-term consequences of AZT therapy will very likely include cancer.

The new recommendation means that the market for AZT will be expanded, despite the fact that individual patients will consume less on a daily basis. This point was made at a noisy annual meeting of Wellcome PLC, the British parent company of Burroughs Wellcome. Sir Alfred Shepperd, the Wellcome chairman, announced that on 29 January 1990 the FDA would recommend whether AZT should be prescribed for symptomless HIV carriers, who are estimated to number up to two million world-wide, as compared to only 200,000 with the full-blown syndrome. Sir Alfred stated:

We are hopeful that within a very short time this drug will be able to play a part in the therapy of a broader group of HIV-infected people. [Reuter dispatch, 16 January 1990]

Thanks to the sales of AZT, which amounted to $225 million last year, the last two years have been very good for Wellcome.   Wellcome made pre-tax profits of $469.4 million in the year to 26 August 1989, on sales of $2.34 billion.   In 1988 Wellcome made pre-tax profits of $367.2 million on sales of $2.08 billion.

However, what's good for Wellcome is not necessarily good for human beings.   At least the FDA is moving in the right direction.   Their new recommendation is halfway to the optimum dose of AZT: none!

#

IX. AZT For Healthy People

An advisory committee of the Food and Drug Administration (FDA) recommended on Tuesday, 30 January 1990, that the use of AZT (or Retrovir) be greatly expanded. At present, AZT is officially recommended only for patients who have T-4 cell counts below 200, or who have been diagnosed as having "AIDS". The committee's recommendation was that AZT be approved for treatment of the estimated one-half million or more people in the United States who have slightly subnormal T-4 cell counts (below 500) and who have antibodies to the human immunodeficiency virus (HIV-1), a retrovirus that is officially, though probably erroneously, considered to be the cause of "AIDS". It is almost always the policy of the FDA to follow the recommendations of its advisory committees.

Actually, many healthy though "positive" gay men are already taking AZT, in the belief that the drug will delay an inevitable progression to "AIDS" (a belief which is not supported by scientific evidence). The new recommendation, if adopted by the FDA, will greatly expand the market for AZT in two ways. First, it would overcome the reluctance many physicians have about prescribing a highly toxic drug for any but desperately sick patients. Second, it would facilitate payment for AZT treatment, currently estimated at $4,000 per year, from Medicaid and from private health insurance plans.

The Antiviral Drugs Advisory Committee reached its decision on the basis of two studies, skimpy and incoherent summations of which were promulgated last summer through government press releases. Allegedly, HIV-positive people given AZT were less likely to develop "AIDS" or to become sick, in ways that were not clearly defined. These "preliminary findings" have not yet been written up, let alone published in a reputable scientific journal. No adequate description of the studies' design and methodology has been published. No hard data are available anywhere. And yet the committee, on the basis of government-industry say-so -- without ever seeing the original (and possibly apocryphal) data -- recommended that a highly toxic drug be given, on a lifetime basis, to people who are perfectly healthy.

The committee seems to have taken a light-minded approach to the extreme toxicity of AZT. The drug can cause life-threatening anemia, severe muscular pain and atrophy, and damage to the liver, kidneys, and nerves. In addition, our best information indicates that long-term use of AZT will result in cancer. Burroughs Wellcome, the manufacturer, recently announced that their drug had caused cancer in rodents. And the results from a standard in vitro test, the Cell Transformation Assay, indicated that AZT should be presumed to be a potential carcinogen. In a half-hearted acknowledgement of these problems, the committee stated:

> While this benefit has been clearly established [not true], the committee emphasized the need to carefully study and document the potential risks associated with prolonged zidovudine therapy, especially those related to the drug's cancer-causing potential, and any possible unique effects on women's fetuses and children. (Quoted in AP press release of 30 January 1990.)

Considering that nothing is known about the long-term effects of AZT therapy, the committee's recommendation is frivolous. No human being has taken AZT for more than three and a half years. Virtually no patients have been able to take what was originally the full dose of AZT, 1200 mg. per day, for more than a few months without requiring transfusions and/or discontinuance of the drug. The acute or short-term toxicities of AZT are horrible enough. The chronic or long-term toxicities have yet to be discovered, and there is no reason to be optimistic.

The Press

Dispatches from the Associated Press and Reuter Information Services were at least sufficiently objective to discuss the issue of AZT's cancer-causing potential. This was not the case with such AIDS-Mob toadies as Gina Kolata and Michael Spector.

Kolata's story in the New York Times (31 January 1990) is written with her customary sloppiness. For instance, she writes: "The agency [FDA] currently recommends that people take AZT once their T-4 counts fall below 200, the point at which they are considered to have AIDS." The CDC's surveillance definition of "AIDS" may have changed several times, but I am not aware that a T-4 cell count below 200 qualifies for an "AIDS" diagnosis.

At some length Kolata mulls over the question of whether a patient on long-term AZT therapy might develop AZT-resistant strains of the "AIDS virus". Nowhere, however, does she broach the far more important issue of AZT's toxicities or its potential to cause cancer. Ignoring such unpleasant things she concludes her account with the sycophantic assertion that "because the drug delays the progress of AIDS it would improve the quality of a patient's life and should be used when T-4 cells drop."

Michael Spector's article in the Washington Post is less flaky, but he also fails to mention the issue of cancer. This is truly amazing. Here is a drug, being recommended for healthy people, with the expectation that they will have to take it for the rest of their lives. The best available information indicates that long-term use of the drug will cause cancer. And reporters like Kolata and Spector don't consider this to be newsworthy.

On the issue of cancer: Would AZT still have been approved by the FDA if the rodent carcinogenicity studies had been finished first, as they were supposed to have been?   Do any of the AIDS journalists even think about such things?

Ramifications For Business
The committee's recommendation doesn't make sense in scientific terms, and it doesn't make sense in human terms.   But in marketing terms, it is right on the mark.   The FDA's decision two weeks ago to recommend cutting the recommended AZT dose in half is clearly part of the same marketing strategy, in which Burroughs Wellcome and the FDA are accomplices. Lowering the dose means that most healthy people would be able to withstand the acute toxicities of AZT, thus making it possible to recommend long-term treatment.   This point was made by Sir Alfred Shepperd, the chairman of Wellcome PLC (the British-based parent company of Burroughs Wellcome) when he announced that on 29 January 1990 the FDA would recommend whether AZT should be prescribed for symptomless HIV-positive people (estimated to number up to two million world-wide, as compared to only 200,000 with the full-blown syndrome).   In the unctuous words of Sir Alfred:

> We are hopeful that within a very short time this drug will be able to play a part in the therapy of a broader group of HIV-infected people. [Reuter dispatch, 16 January 1990]

It is estimated that there are from 500,000 to 650,000 potential customers for AZT in the U.S.--people who are HIV-positive and have T-4 cell counts below 500.   However, there is a serious, though not insuperable, marketing problem here.   Most and perhaps nearly all of these targeted consumers are unaware that they carry antibodies to HIV.   On top of that, they don't feel sick (probably because they are in fact perfectly healthy).   How is Burroughs Wellcome to persuade them to take an expensive drug, with no scientifically established benefits, that will give them violent headaches, destroy their bone marrow, and cause their muscles to shrivel up? How, indeed?

The answer is to conduct a massive propaganda campaign among members of "high risk groups" (meaning primarily us: gay men) to persuade them to take the HIV antibody test. Those who test "positive" will then be counselled to have T-cell tests done regularly, under the care of an enabling physician. Those whose T-4 cells drop below 500 at some point -- whether from a cold, anxiety, or whatever -- will be subjected to further counselling. They will be told that they are suffering from infection with a deadly virus, that their illness is incurable and invariably fatal. However, the "good news" is that AZT will "delay the progression", and that with luck the patient may be able to survive for a number of years. "HIV is a manageable disease" is one of the new slogans.

This campaign has already been going full steam for several months. Such gay quisling groups as Project Inform and Gay Men's Health Crisis, and such writers as Michael Hellquist in the Advocate, have joined the bandwagon. A typical ad is one that appears in the 26 January 1990 issue of the Connecticut magazine, Metroline ("News for the Gay Community").

If the FDA adopts the recommendation of the advisory committee, which it probably will, then most doctors will feel obliged to have their gay male patients tested for HIV antibodies, and if "positive", for T-4 counts. The unfortunate patients who qualify will then be put on AZT. Their health will deteriorate, but always in line with the physician's perception that AZT is "delaying the progression".

The new FDA recommendation will also ensure payment for AZT, through either public or private insurers. If things go as planned, 1990 ought to be a very good year for Wellcome, just as 1989 was. In 1989 worldwide sales of AZT were 225 million dollars, including 148 million dollars in the U.S. alone.

[Below is the ad from Metroline:]

Ramifications For Gay Men

There are estimated to be 40,000 people taking AZT
in the United States.   Most of these are gay men.   For
two and a half years I have been doing my best to
warn of the dangers of AZT, and I have persuaded a
lot of people not to take it.   The fact remains that
tens of thousands of gay men are now taking AZT, and
many tens of thousand more will take it if the FDA
goes through with its new recommendation.   They will
trust their doctors, the "gay leaders", the government,
and Burroughs Wellcome.   It is hard for the mind to
grasp the horror of what is happening.

I do not think the next few years will be good for
us.   A genocidal campaign has been launched against
gay men, with the full collaboration of our gay dupes
and traitors.   The AIDS Mob is trying to poison us,
psychologically and physically.   We've got to fight
back! DON'T TAKE THE TEST!

#

X. A "State Of The Art" AZT Conference
(Or The Banality Of Evil)

Last weekend I travelled to Washington, DC to attend a "State of the Art Conference on AZT Therapy for Early HIV Infection", sponsored by the National Institute of Allergy and Infectious Diseases (NIAID), held in the National Institutes of Health (NIH) head-quarters in Bethesda, Maryland on 3 March 1990. The purpose of the conference was described as follows in a NIAID press release:

> The conference goal is the development of specific recommendations for the use of AZT (zido-vudine) by physicians who care for patients with early HIV infection. A panel of AIDS researchers, community physicians, statisticians, and other experts will review data from clinical trials and other relevant studies of AZT. During the last hour of the meeting opportunities will be provided for questions and comments from the audience.

The timing of the conference coincided fortuitously with a decision of the Food and Drug Administration the day before (2 March 1990) to approve the use of AZT for healthy people having antibodies to the ten-dentiously named human immunodeficiency virus (HIV), also known as the "AIDS virus". With the new recom-mendation, physicians will be encouraged to have their "high risk" patients (like gay men) tested for HIV antibodies, and then to prescribe AZT for those pa-tients who test positive and whose T-4 cells drop below a count of 500 cells per cubic milliliter of blood (a count which is slightly below normal).

A testimonial to the drug was given by no less a public official than Health and Human Services Secre-tary Louis Sullivan, who said:

> The studies and the change in labeling mean that better treatment can now be offered to thousands

of people at earlier stages of infection with the AIDS virus before their health deteriorates critically.[1]

The FDA decision to recommend AZT for long-term use by healthy people goes together with another recent FDA decision to halve the recommended daily dose of AZT to 600 milligrams per day. Prior to the dose reduction, AZT's acute toxicities were so great that few if any patients could take the drug for more than a few months without requiring transfusions, discontinuance of the drug, or both. AZT is now the most toxic drug ever prescribed for long-term use.

The conference consisted mainly of slide talks, accompanied by sometimes desultory discussion. NIAID has promised to furnish a written document on the conference, which I'll review if and when I receive it. In this article I'll describe the general nature of the conference, followed by highlights of individual presentations.

Manipulating Group Consensus

The conclusions of the conference were obviously determined well in advance. The panel of experts, after reviewing data from slide talks, were supposed to bolster the FDA decision of the previous day by recommending to physicians that they should give AZT to HIV positive members of high risk groups with T-4 cell counts below 500.

The panel was stacked, inasmuch as it contained no critics, but many advocates of AZT. The panel members fell into two main segments. The first segment, comprising the majority of panelists, were independents, who were willing to be persuaded one way or another. The other segment consisted of hard-core AZT partisans, players on the Burroughs-Wellcome team

---

[1]"AIDS Drug", Associated Press, 3 March 1990.

(and presumably payroll). The struggle was unequal--as Lenin forcefully demonstrated, both in theory and in practice, a disciplined and surreptitious minority can powerfully prevail against a fragmented and unorganized majority. The independents were concerned with the truth, as well as the welfare of the human beings to whom AZT might be prescribed, and so they were properly hesitant or cautious at times. The AZT partisans had no such inhibitions: they acted in concert, and in line with a clear and pre-determined goal.

My presence was regarded as a threat by the organizers of the conference, and with good reason. I have now written more on AZT than any other writer in the world, and I am one of the very few writers (including Joseph Sonnabend, Peter Duesberg, Celia Farber, Ian Young, Brian Deer, Katie Leishman, and Gary Null) who have dared to expose the lies supporting this deadly nostrum.

For several days before the conference I had carried on discussions with the organizers over whether I could gain admittance to the main conference room, or be relegated to an "overflow room" from which I could "observe the proceedings by closed circuit telecast." They intransigently insisted on the latter. When I arrived at the conference, several tensely officious females were ready and waiting. One of them informed me that an "overflow situation" existed, and that if I even attempted to take a look inside the main room, guards would be called. Another wrote my name on a waiting list. Admitting temporary defeat, I went into the "overflow room", and watched the first three presentations on the television screen. The visual quality was so poor that it was impossible to read the numbers that appeared on the slide tables. Having a view of the door, I could see person after person being admitted into the main room, even two hours after the conference had begun. Then, during the mid-morning break, one of my colleagues, who had simply walked into the main room, informed me that, far from an "overflow situation", there were at least three dozen empty seats. With a rush of adrenalin, I gathered up my gear and walked into the main room. No one attempted to stop me, and for the rest of the day I was able to observe live human beings presenting legible (if sometimes dubious) information.

Slide talks are, by their very nature, a form of propaganda. It is almost impossible to comprehend, evaluate, and retain the data that are flashed on the screen. One cannot, as when reading a detailed written report, dig in, go back and forth over methodology, tables, graphs, etc. Instead, information washes over one, the critical faculties are dulled, and one ends up accepting the generalities and conclusions that are offered by the presenter.

In spite of the one-sided planning of the conference, the desired consensus was not reached, and a couple of bombshells went off. Before going into highlights of the presentations, I'd like to give credit to Charles C.J. Carpenter, Professor of Medicine at Brown University, who did a good job of chairing the conference. Carpenter was fair and impartial, and did his best to maintain standards of civility among the panelists.

Margaret Fischl

Margaret Fischl is one of the stars on the Burroughs-Wellcome team. She coordinated the fraud-ridden Phase II AZT trials, which I analyzed two and a half years ago.[2] When I spoke to Fischl on a previous occasion, she was unable to answer some very simple questions about a report which she herself had alleged-

_____

[2]Native Issue 235. Another highly critical review of the Phase II trials was written by Joseph A. Sonnabend, "Review of AZT Multicenter Trial Data Obtained Under the Freedom of Information Act by Project Inform and ACT-UP", AIDS Forum, January 1988.

ly written, and she referred me to Burroughs Wellcome for answers. It is scandalous that someone of her caliber should have been allowed to supervise clinical trials in the first place, let alone to continue to do so.

Fischl's first slide talk was on "NIAID AIDS Clinical Trials Group Protocol 016: The Safety and Efficacy of AZT in the Treatment of Patients with Early ARC." In this study patients with "early ARC" were treated with AZT, and allegedly remained in better health than did patients who received a placebo. When I commented on this study last August, I wrote:

> The study design was rotten at its core through sheer subjectivity. The "exciting" results were based entirely on perceived progressions from milder to more serious symptoms -- on progressions from gray to gray. If no one at NIAID even knew what the qualifying symptoms were, one can only imagine the cognitive chaos that must have prevailed in the field, when physicians had to decide if a particular configuration of symptoms qualified as mild ARC, serious ARC, AIDS, or none of these.[3]

Nothing in Fischl's presentation shed light on this central problem. Interestingly, much of the claimed efficacy of AZT in this study was based on results from the now-discredited p-24 antigen test, about which more later.

Fischl blithely dismissed AZT's toxicities by claiming the drug was "remarkably well tolerated". Although fatigue, malaise, nausea, and hematologic abnormalities were found more frequently in the AZT than in the placebo group, almost all patients taking a low dose were able to tolerate the drug -- according to Fischl.

Margaret Fischl later gave a second slide talk, entitled "NIAID AIDS Clinical Trials Group Protocol 002: The Safety and Efficacy of AZT in the Treatment

---

[3]Native Issue 331.

of Patients with Post First Episode PCP." Fischl said this was a brand new study: "I almost feel like the birth of a baby!" (No, I am not kidding. She really did say that.) The point of this study was to compare the efficacy of a low dose (600 mg./day) with that of a high dose (1200 mg./day) of AZT in patients who had had one episode of pneumocystis carinii pneumonia (PCP). Apparently the low dose was just as effective as the high dose, and with less hematologic toxicity.

On the whole, AZT did not do a very good job of "extending the lives" of the patients in Protocol 002. After two years of treatment, 66 to 72 percent of them were dead.

No report has been written or published on either of these studies. I refuse to comment on them further until I can look at a proper report in a peer-reviewed journal. From a complete written report an analyst can analyze methodology, study design, or data -- but he cannot analyze the generalities and snippets of information that are tossed out in a slide talk. Based on Fischl's past record, no research in which she has taken part should be accepted without considerable skepticism.

Paul Volberding

Paul Volberding from San Francisco was another of the Burroughs-Wellcome stars. His talk, dually presented with Stephen Lagakos of the Harvard School of Public Health, was entitled, "NIAID AIDS Clinical Trials Group Protocol 019: The Safety and Efficacy of AZT for Asymptomatic HIV Infected Individuals." This, of course, was the theme of the conference. The alleged results from Protocol 019 had previously been promulgated in a skimpy and incoherent NIAID press release on 17 August 1989. At the time I characterized this practice as "The great AZT scam: results without data".[4]

Allegedly, HIV positive individuals on either a low or a high dose of AZT were less likely to develop AIDS than were those on placebo.   Unfortunately, Volberding and Lagakos did not present sufficient data to support this conclusion.

However, a number of interesting statements were made during their presentations.   One of the patients was murdered during the course of the study.   Volberding admitted to a "strong suspicion" that most of the patients knew whether they were getting AZT of placebo.   The "suspicion" was strengthened by the fact that patients on placebo were far more likely to drop out of the study.   In other words, the study was not really blind, as it was designed to be!   The study was therefore invalid on this basis alone.

Stephen Lagakos gave an excruciatingly inept performance.   The numbers he presented were illegible on the television screen I was watching at the time.   However, he showed a line chart depicting CD4 counts over time by treatment group.   A glance was enough to show that there was no clear pattern, and the differences were trivial.   This is what he should have said.   But instead he talked endlessly about a meaningless chart.

During a break Volberding told me that a report on Protocol 019 was "in the process of being reviewed", and that he hoped it would be published soon.   Fine.   When I see the report I'll comment on this research further.[5]

----

[4]Native Issue 340.

[5]The article was published just as this book is going to press. Paul A. Volberding, Stephen W. Lagakos, et al., "Zidovudine in Asymptomatic Human Im-
(continued...)

Since Volberding and Lagakos, as well as Fischl, frequently made reference to results on the p-24 antigen test, as a measure of AZT's efficacy, a brief discussion on this topic is in order.

The Discredited P-24 Antigen Test: A Digression

As readers of the Native are aware, the p-24 antigen test is unvalidated -- it is not known exactly what the test measures, or how accurately it measures it. Over two years ago, Harvey Bialy, Research Editor of Bio/Technology, wrote an editorial in which he assailed the uncritical use of the test, the shoddy peer-review standards of medical journals, and the gullibility of the press.[6] Bialy demonstrated that the claimed results from the p-24 antigen test, as reported in recent medical journals, could not possibly be true.

---

[5](...continued)
munodeficiency Virus Infection: A Controlled Trial in Persons with Fewer than 500 CD4-Positive Cells per Cubic Millimeter", New England Journal of Medicine, 5 April 1990.

In brief, the research is unacceptable. The authors' ignorance of elementary statistics is beyond belief. None of their tables show bases or make sense. Willy-nilly they compare percents with raw numbers.

Much of the article consists of crude special pleading. As support for the "benefits" of AZT, the authors cite the fraudulent Phase II Trials (Chapter II) and the shoddy AZT survival study (Chapter V), along with the ridiculous Pizzo study (p. 21). However, they don't even mention the far superior Dournon study (p. 138).

In no way does this article demonstrate benefits of AZT treatment for asymptomatic, HIV-infected persons.

[6]Harvey Bialy, "Commentary: Where is the Virus? And Where is the Press?", Bio/Technology, February 1988.

A year later the eminent molecular biologist, Peter Duesberg, in his magisterial refutation of the hypothesis that HIV is the cause of "AIDS", demonstrated the worthlessness of the p-24 antigen test, pointing out that, among other things:

All studies on p24 report AIDS cases that occur without p24 antigenemia, indicating that p24 is not necessary for AIDS.   They also report antigenemia without AIDS, indicating that p24 is not sufficient for AIDS.[7]

In the 14 December 1989 issue of the New England Journal of Medicine, two articles and an editorial appeared, which attempted to show that, contrary to the arguments of Duesberg, HIV really is biochemically active, and therefore might still be either a cause or the cause of "AIDS".   Both articles demonstrated that results from the p-24 antigen test were meaningless.[8] In an editorial, David Baltimore wrote:

If this new approach [to drug testing] is to succeed, accurate early markers of drug efficacy will be of great value.   None of the currently available "surrogate" markers are completely satisfactory in this regard.   Detectable quantities of p24 antigen are found in only a fraction of infected persons and, as shown by Ho and Coombs and their

---

[7] Peter H. Duesberg, Human Immunodeficiency Virus and Acquired Immunodeficiency Syndrome: Correlation But Not Causation", Proceedings of the National Academy of Sciences, February 1989.

[8] David D. Ho et al., "Quantitation of Human Immunodeficiency Virus Type 1 in the Blood of Infected Persons", New England Journal of Medicine, 14 December 1989.
   Robert W. Coombs et al., "Plasma Viremia in Human Immunodeficiency Virus Infection", ibid.

coworkers, correlate poorly with the presence or amount of replicating HIV.[9]

My point, then, is that much of the AZT research for the past three years has relied upon results from the p-24 antigen test -- a test which is now admitted, even by advocates of the HIV hypothesis, to be worthless.

A digression within a digression: The New England Journal of Medicine has agreed to run a letter from Peter Duesberg replying to the articles by Ho, Coombs, Baltimore, and Feinberg. In scientific, as opposed to propagandistic terms, the HIV hypothesis has not yet risen from the grave.

John D. Hamilton

The major bombshell of the conference was detonated by John D. Hamilton, a soft-spoken gentleman who is Professor of Medicine at Duke University. His talk was entitled, "Veterans Administration Study #298: AZT Treatment of AIDS and ARC, Part I: Treatment of Patients with ARC." This was a large case-control study evaluating AZT treatment (1500 mg./day) of patients whose T-4 counts were between 200 and 500. The principal endpoints were AIDS, death, or both.

Although Hamilton was not able to release specific data, owing to a rule which some medical journals have (if data from a study have been made public, the article is automatically rejected), he did give the major conclusions. Whether looking at survival, clinical benefits, quality of life, or any other measure, there was no evidence that AZT had benefits of any kind.

Hamilton's conclusion, understated but authoritative, was this:

---

[9]David Baltimore and Mark B. Feinberg, "HIV Revealed: Toward a Natural History of the Infection", ibid.

In conclusion: We hope this panel will acknowledge the uncertainties discussed today, and that the message to patients and practitioners will reflect the lack of information in many areas.

This was the last thing the Burroughs-Wellcome Mob wanted to hear. Why should a physician prescribe a toxic drug for long-term use if the drug has no benefits at all? Several times as Hamilton was speaking, Margaret Fischl, whether from nervousness or boorishness, went into episodes of snickering. This may be her mode of refutation. Over two years ago, when I asked her if she had read Peter Duesberg's article in Cancer Research refuting the HIV hypothesis, she responded by snickering.

Under sharp questioning from the AZT advocates, Hamilton expressed confidence in his study, which was carefully designed and had large samples. He considered it most unlikely that the results would change appreciably over time.

Mitchell Gail

The most ludicrous presentation of the conference was given by Mitchell Gail, a "Medical Statistical Investigator" with the National Cancer Institute (NCI): "Recent Deficits in the Incidence of AIDS". He tried to make the utterly preposterous case that AZT therapy should be given credit for the fact that the incidence of AIDS is going down.

Well now, I have been arguing for three years that the CDC projections of AIDS incidence were far too high.[10] I demonstrated a year and a half ago that the incidence of AIDS was dropping.[11] Until just recently public health service officials simply denied all this--

---

[10]Native Issue 203.

[11]Native Issue 286.

they said that the estimates were accurate and the incidence was not dropping. However, it is now clear that the CDC projections for 1988 and 1989 were far too high, and everyone wants an explanation (as though it were not in the nature of epidemics to peak at some point).

Whatever the explanation may be, it cannot be AZT, which has only recently been given to small numbers of "asymptomatic" people.

AZT and Cancer

Kenneth Ayers, Senior Toxicologist at Burroughs Wellcome, spoke on "AZT Carcinogenicity". He discussed the recent rodent carcinogenicity studies, in which AZT caused vaginal tumors in mice and rats. Ayers did a competent job of presenting the findings, although, being on the payroll of Burroughs-Wellcome, he tended to downplay their significance.

Some of his information went beyond that which was available last December, when I reported on these findings.[12]   For example, back in December apologists for AZT, such as James Mason of the Public Health Service or Mathilde Krim of AmFAR, claimed that the AZT doses given the rodents were far higher than the equivalent human doses. I argued at the time that this could not be true, since at such high doses the rodents would all have perished from anemia. Now it turns out that the information given in the press had been quite incomplete. In both rodent studies, the doses of AZT had to be sharply reduced "in the interest of long-term survival". In the study on rats, the doses were reduced sharply after 90 days, and had to be reduced even further after 279 days.

Ayers explored the question of how AZT causes vaginal cancer in rodents, and inclined to the hypothesis that cancer results from local contact of vaginal

---

[12]Native Issue 348.

tissue with urine with high AZT concentration. Interestingly, rodents absorb much less AZT than do
human beings. Whereas rodent excrete 90% of the AZT
they are given, humans excrete only 20%. Therefore,
the systemic, as opposed to localized, toxicities of AZT
may be much worse in humans than in rodents.

Ayers correctly stated that the significance of the
rodent carcinogenicity studies was: an indication of
general carcinogenic risk in humans. He then went on
to characterize AZT as a weak rather than a general
carcinogen, and to claim that "there are other drugs
that cause cancer in animals, but are still in common
use at the discretion of the physician and the patient."
He failed to mention what those drugs might be, and
whether they are prescribed for long-term use in
healthy people.

Amazingly, Ayers did not even mention the results
of the Cell Transformation Assay, which was performed
over three years ago. In this standard in vitro test
utilizing human cells, AZT proved to be highly positive,
indicating, in the words of the FDA toxicology analyst,
that AZT should be "presumed to be a potential carcinogen". Burroughs-Wellcome is well aware of this
finding, as it is alluded to (if cryptically) in the AZT
(Retrovir) entry in the Physician's Desk Reference. In
a conference devoted to evaluating the merits of long-
term AZT therapy, in a presentation devoted to "AZT
Carcinogenicity", the failure to discuss or even mention
the Cell Transformation Assay is deplorable, and can
only be regarded as a deliberate intent to deceive on
the part of Burroughs-Wellcome.

Douglas Richman

Douglas Richman from San Diego is also on the
Burroughs-Wellcome team, having been a principal
investigator in the Phase II trials. However, his
presentation, "AZT Resistance", was not very encour-
aging for the AZT advocates. In brief, he reported
that HIV does develop resistance to AZT over time,

and there are many unanswered questions in this area. Obviously, for those who believe that HIV is the cause of "AIDS", such resistance would not bode well for long-term therapy.

Discussion Among the Panel

Most of the afternoon was devoted to discussion on various topics among the panel. Jay Sanford, President and Dean of the Uniformed Services University of the Health Sciences, made a key point: If the progression rate (from HIV infection with low T-4 counts to AIDS) is so low anyway (4% or less), is it really justified to give AZT on a mass scale? None of the AZT advocates attempted to answer him.

Neil Schram, a gay physician from Palos Verdes, California, emphasized that hasty decisions (like taking AZT) should not be made on a single CD4 count, as such readings normally go up and down in the course of a day, and transient infections like flu can greatly lower the CD4 counts. He added that many patients look upon their CD4 counts in absolute terms, and are unaware of the expected day-to-day and hour-to-hour variance in these readings.

On the topic, "Monitoring of Patient Immune Status", the p-24 antigen test was described as having no practical value by three of the panel members. No one defended the test.

In the discussion, "Initiation of AZT Therapy", Neil Schram dissented from the encroaching consensus that AZT should be given to all HIV positive individuals with T-4 counts below 500. He said he didn't know-- that the Veterans Administration study had changed his mind, and he was no longer willing to say that AZT should be given to those with T-4 counts between 200 and 500. Schram's caution was impermissible, and immediately he came under attack from Fischl and Volberding. Fischl characterized Schram's hesitation as "dangerous", and said that "We must rely on the data before us" (meaning presumably the unpublished data from Volberding and herself). Anthony Fauci then entered the fray, siding with Fischl and Volberding against Schram. According to Fauci, those who start AZT earlier (when their counts are higher) do better than those who start AZT later.

This was rather an ugly episode, and I think that homophobia played a role in the contempt with which three straights (Fischl, Volberding, and Fauci) addressed a gay man. Fortunately other panel members came to Schram's defense — Robert Couch, Professor and Chairman of the Department of Microbiology and Immunology at the Baylor College of Medicine, pointedly told the AZT gang that Neil Schram was not the only one with misgivings over the blanket recommendation. Jay Sanford and Gerald Friedland, Professor of Medicine and Epidemiology and Social Medicine at the Albert Einstein College of Medicine, also supported the caution of Schram and Couch. Fischl responded by pleading with the panel to "Give the positive message" (presumably meaning to recommend AZT).

The discussion, "The Management of HIV Infected Individuals on AZT Therapy", was largely concerned with what to do about the toxic side effects of AZT: anemia, neutropenia, myopathy (a muscular disorder), etc. Here the discussion became very unreal: whether to reduce doses, or to discontinue therapy; whether to resume therapy, and at what doses, and so on. To pose such a question is to answer it: What should be done if the administration of a toxic drug has caused a patient to become anemic, or his muscles to ache violently and shrivel up? How much common sense does it take to make a decision?

Public Discussion

As time was running short, only a half hour was available for public discussion. I put my name in early, and ought to have been the third person in line. However, a woman deposited more slips of paper on the Chairman's podium, and then Anthony Fauci went up and rearranged the slips. With about five minutes to go, it didn't look as though I would be allowed to speak, so I went up to the podium and explained to Charles Carpenter that I thought I was next. I found the slip with my name on it on the bottom of the pile, and handed it to him. He then called on me, and I introduced myself and said something like the following:

I'd like to express my concern in two areas. First, caution is needed regarding the chronic toxicities of AZT. We do not know what the long-term side effects of this drug are in human beings. We should not minimize the potential of AZT to cause cancer. I was shocked that the toxicologist from Burroughs-Wellcome did not even mention the results of the Cell Transformation Assay, which was performed well over three years ago. In that standard in vitro test of carcinogenicity, involving human cells, AZT was found to be highly positive. The results mean, in the words of an FDA toxicologist, that "AZT should be presumed to be a potential carcinogen." Burroughs-Wellcome is well aware of these results, as a reference to them appears in the Retrovir entry in the Physician's Desk Reference.

Second, skepticism is needed regarding unpublished data purporting to show benefits of AZT. For one thing, there are studies that show no long-term benefits of AZT therapy. A case-control study conducted in France by Dournon and colleagues found that the very, very slight "benefits" of AZT vanished and were utterly nonexistent after six months.[13]   And today we have heard that a Veter-

---

[13]E. Dournon et al., "Effects of Zidovudine [AZT] in 365 Consecutive Patients With AIDS or AIDS-Related Complex", The Lancet, 3 December 1988.

an's Administration study found no benefits at all from AZT therapy.

In addition, we need to be skeptical because many of the studies allegedly demonstrating AZT's benefits were very bad research. I've done an analysis of the Phase II trials, which were the basis for AZT's approval, using documents the FDA was forced to release under the Freedom of Information Act. In that study, sloppiness and cheating of all kinds was tolerated. Among the many sins that were committed against the ethics of science, the investigators deliberately used data that they knew were false. Only one word is adequate to describe such "research". That word is FRAUD.

Conclusions

The AZT conference enhanced my appreciation of Hannah Arendt's phrase, the "banality of evil". Most of the participants in the conference were not intrinsically evil. Some of them were weak, conformist, susceptible to peer pressure or bribery. But the majority were good people doing their best to make fair and rational decisions based on the information available to them.

Nevertheless, the panel members were leading players in a monumentally evil program -- the terrorizing and poisoning of gay men and other members of "risk groups". Many thousands of people may die because of the actions of the panel, coupled with the FDA decision of the previous day to recommend AZT for healthy people.

Evil people do exist, and some of them were present at the conference -- people whose unchecked egocentrism has made them indifferent or even hostile to the welfare of their fellow human beings. But for the most part, the triumph of evil follows when good people remain silent.

#

XI. Excerpt From Interview With Peter Duesberg [1]
13 June 1987

John Lauritsen: In New York I know one person who's in a terrible dilemma. He knows many other PWAs in New York, who have told him that, according to the grapevine, AZT is poison -- that most patients treated with AZT feel worse, contrary to the propaganda, and that there are terrible side effects.

Peter Duesberg: It is a poison. It is cytotoxic.

JL: His doctor has insisted he go on AZT.[2] Considering that it's not proven that HIV -- or for that matter any virus -- is the cause of AIDS, what is the good of giving AIDS patients this kind of treatment?

PD: AZT? Well, to put it as kindly as possible, I think it's highly irresponsible. I could go further. Even if the virus were the cause of the disease, the only time that AZT could possibly interfere with the infection would be during the phase when the virus makes DNA. The AZT is an inhibitor of DNA. So in effect it could be like a "morning after" pill -- if you knew you were infected the night before, and took the AZT, you might have a chance of hitting the virus. But it also hits all other DNA that is made. It is hell for the bone marrow, which is where the T and B cells are made. It's hell for that. It has a slight preference for viral DNA polymerase, compared to cellular DNA polymerase, based on in vitro studies only, but that's certainly not absolute. It kills normal cells

---

[1] Native Issue 220.

[2] The person did go on AZT, and died less than a year later.

quite, quite extensively. And considering the size of the target -- the normal cells are so much bigger than the virus -- even if AZT has a preference for the virus, you will hurt the normal cells no end. That's guaranteed. That you hurt the virus is rather hypothetical. Certainly by the time a patient has symptoms of the disease, given the long latent period of the disease, and given the fact that the virus is inactive even in the acute form of the disease, I see no rationale for treating with AZT. Considering that the virus has already been in an AIDS patient for five years, and there's no evidence that it's making DNA at that time, I think that giving AZT is highly irresponsible.

There was a talk here two months ago, and the speaker couldn't explain the rationale for treating with AZT. He didn't know. So I said, "Why don't you use aspirin?" And everybody laughed. He had no answer. He got mad at me. He is a doctor, ministering to the sick, seeing people die, and doesn't understand the basis for it all.

JL: I understand there are almost no data on AZT. The double-blind study was prematurely aborted after only five and a half months. They have not even tracked the people from that study who are still taking AZT, so we have no idea what percentage of them are still alive. They have no data on what percentages of patients suffer from specific side effects.

PD: There are not even any good animal studies. Later they claimed results from mice that were treated first and then inoculated with the virus. There it clearly has an effect. But that's when you get high virus titers and you know you're shooting up now. But five years later? There's no basis for doing so, because the DNA is made by then. The virus is just sitting there and making RNA from existing DNA. And the drug is only going to hurt you.

#

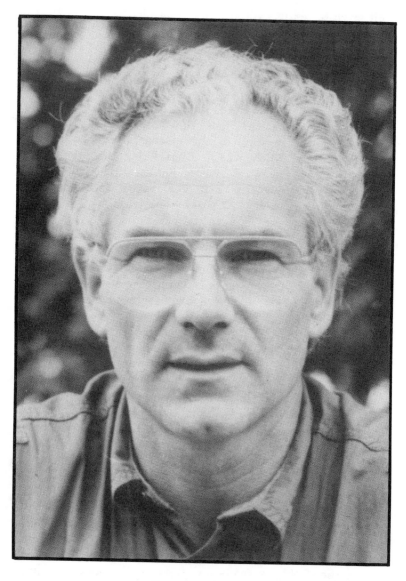

Peter Duesberg
Professor of Molecular Biology, Berkeley
Photograph June 1987 by John Lauritsen

XII. Kangaroo Court Etiology

A "Scientific Forum on the Etiology of AIDS", sponsored by the American Foundation for AIDS Research (AmFAR), was held on 9 April 1988 at the George Washington University in Washington, D.C. In the words of the AmFAR "fact sheet", the Forum was "convened to critically examine the evidence that human immunodeficiency virus (HIV) or other agents give rise to the disease complex known as AIDS. Data from laboratory, clinical, and epidemiological research will be presented and evaluated. The forum seeks no consensus, instead it is designed to permit discussion among experts on the conclusions the facts permit."

As one of the 17 journalists who were privileged to attend, I looked forward to the forum as the first opportunity for an open discussion of the pros and cons of the hypothesis that HIV is the cause of AIDS. Ever since Secretary Heckler announced in 1984 that the cause of AIDS had been discovered, HIV has been accepted as the cause in the absence of any convincing proof that it is. The Public Health Service and the rest of the medical establishment have acquiesced in a "Proof by Proclamation". The forum offered the first opportunity for Peter Duesberg, Professor of Molecular Biology at the University of California at Berkeley, to confront members of the "AIDS establishment" over their HIV hypothesis. (Readers of the Native are aware that over a year ago Duesberg provided a comprehensive and cogently argued refutation of the HIV hypothesis, and that the "AIDS establishment" has intransigently refused to reply to his critique.[1])

Despite these praiseworthy intentions, the forum appears to have had a hidden agenda: to discredit Duesberg. Even Michael Specter, a reporter who

---

[1] Native Issue 220.

toadies to the "AIDS establishment" and is bitterly opposed to Duesberg, admitted that the April 9 meeting "was billed as a scientific forum on the cause of AIDS but was really an attempt to put Duesberg's theories to rest."[2]

The forum represented several steps forward, and several backward. At least the ice has been broken, and the causes of AIDS are now an acceptable topic for public discussion. While no blows were struck, some of the HIV protagonists fell below the standards of civility that are expected in scholarly debate. Nothing particularly new was said, and there was little of the give and take that characterize genuine scientific dialogue. At the same time, the positions of both sides have become more sharply defined; it is now clear what directions future debate should take.

On the whole, I regard the forum as a victory for Duesberg. The forum was a well-orchestrated media event, heavily stacked against him, and he took a lot of abuse. Nevertheless, he stood by his guns; he did not recant (as he apparently was expected to); and to the more discerning participants, he exposed the bankruptcy of the arguments currently advanced in favor of the HIV hypothesis. At all times Duesberg retained good manners and a sense of humor, in the face of invective, insults, and clowning from his opponents.

Before going into what each of the panelists said, I'd like to discuss a couple of general issues which came to the fore: Koch's Postulates and the nature of scientific evidence.

Koch's Postulates

The forum was haunted by the specter of Robert Koch, and the postulates that he formulated for "establishing the specificity of a pathogenic micro-or-

---

[2]Michael Specter, "Panel Rebuts Biologist's Claims on Cause of AIDS", Washington Post, 10 April 1988.

ganism". For a century, medical science has used Koch's postulates as the standards for proving that a particular micro-organism causes a particular disease. The first Postulate requires that the microbe be found in all cases of the disease; the second, that the microbe, having been grown in pure culture, be injected into susceptible animals with the result that the same disease is produced; and the third, that the microbial agent create the disease upon transfer from animals made ill by inoculation.

Duesberg has taken the position that Koch's first Postulate should be amended in a conservative direction, so that the microbe must not only be present in all cases, but must also be biochemically active to a clinically relevant degree. His rationale is that present-day technology makes it possible to see viruses that would have remained unknown and undetectable only ten years ago. It is now possible to identify a virus that is present in only one in 100,000 T-cells. So it is not enough to detect a microbe; it must be proven that the microbe is doing something harmful, and to a sufficient degree, that illness results. Duesberg has also commented, that if Koch's first Postulate is not satisfied, there is no need to bother about the remaining postulates.

The HIV advocates, on the other hand, now wish to revise Koch's in a more permissive direction: it would no longer be necessary to find the microbe in all cases of the disease. Mere correlations between microbial antibodies and the progression of the disease would be sufficient. HIV could be proved "epidemiologically" to be the cause of AIDS.

Actually, the HIV advocates talked out of both sides of their mouths with regard to Koch's postulates. On the one hand, they disparaged them as in need of "modification" (read: abandonment); on the other hand, they were doing their best to come up with data that would satisfy at least the first postulate, which is troublesome because it amounts to good common sense.

Public Vs. Private Facts

Duesberg has based his critique of the HIV hypothesis on a thorough review of the published literature on AIDS. In the course of the debate, it appeared that the HIV advocates are trying to shore up their arguments by revising the facts, particularly with regard to the crucial questions of whether or not HIV is ever biochemically active in people with AIDS (PWAs), and whether or not HIV can be detected in all PWAs.

Several times Duesberg was accused by Anthony Fauci and William Haseltine of having based his arguments on research that was "out of date". Duesberg replied that some of the key figures he cited had been used recently by members of the AIDS establishment, and that he looked forward to reading reports of any new data.

A fundamental difference in philosophy is involved here, one which needs to be articulated. On several occasions Duesberg and his supporter, Harry Rubin, asked Fauci or Haseltine for references to back up assertions they had made, and they were rudely rebuffed. Both Duesberg and Rubin belong to the old school, according to which facts are not entirely "real" until they have been published. Scientists are expected to make their data available, together with a detailed description of methodology, so that other scientists, working independently, could attempt to replicate the experiments and verify the results. Science is thus a public activity, where scientists check out each other's work in a mutual endeavor to establish the truth.

Unfortunately, government scientists and others in the AIDS establishment have sometimes been motivated by considerations other than the truth. In the interests of profit, prestige, and public relations, they have resorted to secrecy and deception. A case in point is the well-documented episode in which Robert Gallo attempted to steal credit from the French for the discovery of the "AIDS virus".[3]

The difference in philosophy needs to be emphasized. Duesberg, basing his arguments on public facts, was countered by Fauci and Haseltine, who referred to their own private facts. Now, it is possible that Duesberg's public facts may be wrong, and that Haseltine's and Fauci's private facts may be correct. But even if that were the case, it would be a grave injustice to Duesberg to criticize him for having used public information. When Duesberg insists upon references, he is not quibbling; he is acting in the best tradition of science.

Harold Ginsberg

The panel was moderated by Harold Ginsberg, Professor of Medicine and Microbiology at Columbia University. He began by saying that recording of the forum would not be permitted, although there would be an official transcript of the proceedings, and that the purpose of the forum was to "discuss in an informal and friendly manner the etiology of AIDS." He then went into a presentation of his own. After conceding that "the pathogenesis of HIV is still pretty much a black box", he discussed the characteristics of several viral diseases, including influenza, poliomyelitis, measles, herpes simplex, and hepatitis B. He emphasized that neutralizing antibodies could be present when disease occurs, and did not necessarily prevent viruses from being present in the blood.

Ginsberg's comments served to set the stage against Duesberg by toppling a straw dummy representing selective statements, torn out of context, which Duesberg had made on antibodies. It became obvious that the forum would not favor free and impartial discussion of the issues -- an impartial discussion, after all,

---

[3]The New Scientist, 12 February 1987.

requires an impartial moderator. It was also obvious that the HIV protagonists would employ information overload as a propaganda technique. While Ginsberg's comments were true enough, so far as they went, they were mostly irrelevant to the central issues of the debate. Nevertheless, they conveyed the impression that a vast body of knowledge argued against Duesberg's critique of the HIV hypothesis. Novice reporters, straining to take in all of Ginsberg's information (without the aid of tape recorders), ended up with little space in their heads for the relevant issues.

Marcel Beluda

The next speaker was Marcel Beluda, Professor of Pathology at the University of California at Los Angeles. His presentation dealt with the complex structure and reproduction cycles of retroviruses, and what rules a retrovirus would have to follow in order to cause disease. He said that, with regard to Koch's first Postulate, retroviral DNA should be present in 100% of the cases, and that it was a serious weakness in identifying HIV as the etiological agent that this requirement could not be satisfied.

Beluda's presentation was complex and highly nuanced, and he ran out of time. Nevertheless, his concluding statement came out clear and strong: "We must resolve the 'black box' HIV biological phenomenon."

Harry Rubin

Harry Rubin, Professor of Molecular Biology at the University of California at Berkeley, was one of the pioneers in the field of retrovirology. Twenty years ago Rubin was king of the field; he trained many of the scientists who are today the world's leading retrovirologists.

Rather than discussing the intricacies of molecular biology, which he was as qualified to do as anyone, Rubin went instead to the heart of the matter: the conceptual problems of AIDS. Rubin said that he was disturbed by the simplicity of the causal explanation that had been put forward. An enormous complexity of disease states constitute the AID Syndrome; no fewer than 20 different diseases are classified as "AIDS". Cartesian reductionism -- the notion that complex phenomena can be reduced to a single cause -- didn't make much sense in this context. The simplistic notion of a single disease entity caused by a single virus ignored the role played by the condition of the host -- the complex, life-long interaction between the host, the environment, and microbes.

For Rubin a red flag went up when he learned that Burkitt's lymphoma was classified along with the many other manifestations of AIDS. He recalled that for many years attempts had been made to explain Burkitt's lymphoma and other cancers in terms of viruses, with such candidates as Epstein-Barr virus proposed. The generally favored explanation came to be chromosomal abnormalities. And now, apparently, "HIV infection" is supposed to be a cause of some cancers.

Rubin said that the simplistic HIV causal explanation raised a lot of questions, and recalled a theory that was popular 20 years ago to explain the origin of cancer. The "immune surveillance theory" held that the body somehow lost its immune capacity and, in consequence, its ability to hold down cancers. The theory is no longer talked about owing to experiments on a-thymic mice, known as "nude mice". (Lacking thymus glands, nude mice cannot manufacture T-cells, and therefore lack a cellular immune system.) What dissolved the "immune surveillance theory" was the discovery that nude mice, while susceptible to many different diseases, had no higher incidences of any cancer than did mice with normal immune systems. So, Rubin asked, how can we talk about "immune deficiency" as being responsible for the cancers that are considered to be part of the syndrome known as "AIDS"?

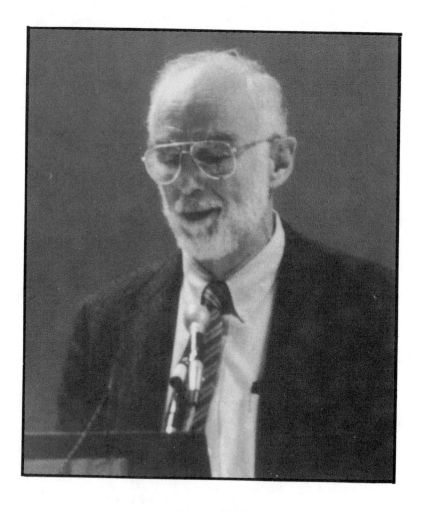

Harry Rubin
Professor of Molecular Biology
University of California, Berkeley
April 1988
Photograph by John Lauritsen

Rubin concluded by saying that he found any single cause of the enormous complex of diseases to be seriously inadequate. While he was not willing categorically to rule out the possibility that HIV might play some role in some cases, he was "not ready blandly to accept it as the single cause of all of the disease complex." Rubin posed the question, to what extent is the virus itself an opportunistic infection? He found it irresponsible to focus exclusive attention on the putative viral cause while failing to address the associated practices of high risk groups (heavy use of recreational drugs, overuse of antibiotics, promiscuous sexual behavior) which are themselves known to compromise the immune system.

In the question period following Rubin's presentation, William Haseltine bluntly challenged Rubin on the issue of high-risk behavior, and asserted that the best correlation with AIDS is "evidence of viral infection", and that there were many instances of AIDS in persons with no known risk factors. Rubin replied that the serological evidence seemed to argue against HIV, since in many PWAs neither antibodies nor virus could be detected.

Beluda then intervened, apparently annoyed by Haseltine's belligerence, to state that sometimes even a single exception is sufficient to disprove a theory. HIV antibodies are reportedly found in 90% of PWAs, but what about the other 10%? "This is the crux of the matter", Beluda said, "the virus cannot be found in all cases of AIDS."

Fauci responded to Beluda by saying that a good lab was able to isolate the virus in 90-100% of the cases, that there was "no question about it". Fauci did not provide a reference to published data, nor did he indicate what the "good labs" were, or how exactly they differed from the not-so-good labs.

Peter Duesberg

Since Duesberg's presentation covered a lot of ground, I'll try to summarize just the main points here. To understand the full scope of his arguments, his latest article should be consulted.[4]

Basically Duesberg argued that HIV does not have the physical properties to cause disease, let alone the devastating pathology associated with AIDS. The HIV hypothesis is fraught with contradictions (or "paradoxes"); it violates the rules that all other microbes follow when they cause disease; indeed, the hypothesis sometimes violates the principle of causality itself.

Duesberg began by attacking the prevailing hypothesis: that HIV kills T-cells after a bizarre latent period of 5-8 years. This cannot be true, he said, because retroviruses do not kill cells -- in fact, retroviruses make cells grow faster. The "AIDS virus" hypothesis is now the basis for over $1 billion research efforts annually, making it the most expensive virus in history. The HIV hypothesis is the basis for the "AIDS test", which is in fact only a test for HIV antibodies. Antibodies, which for 200 years have been interpreted as good news, are now interpreted as a prognosis for death. Positive results on the antibody test have resulted in suicides and broken marriages; they would be the basis for denying residence in China. The presence of HIV antibodies is now being used to justify treatment with AZT, which has one known effect: to stop DNA synthesis; the obligatory consequence of incorporating AZT into a human cell is either a dead or a mutated cell.

The "AIDS virus" hypothesis is based only on correlation -- between HIV antibodies and AIDS -- a

---

[4]Peter Duesberg, "Human Immunodeficiency Virus and Acquired Immunodeficiency Syndrome: Correlation But Not Causation", Proceedings of the National Academy of Sciences, Vol. 86, February 1989.

correlation in the neighborhood of 80-90% ("They never say 100%"). And even if the correlation were 100%, this would not prove causality. Further, antibodies are not the same as the virus itself, which is so extremely difficult to detect that only the most expensive laboratories in the country are capable of doing so, and even then, only in about half of the cases of AIDS.

All known viruses (polio, hepatitis, et al.) are biochemically active when they cause disease. They have to kill or intoxicate more cells than the host can regenerate. Paradoxically: HIV is inactive and latent, even in patients who are dying from AIDS. A virus cannot cause harm without doing something. Although viruses can go through periods of latency, neither herpes nor any other virus is inactive at the time that it causes disease. HIV actively infects fewer than one in 10,000 T-cells, even in fatal cases of AIDS. This is trivial, the equivalent of losing one drop of blood every day.

Viruses cause disease before, not after antiviral immunity. This is why vaccination works. Paradoxically: HIV is said to cause AIDS only after a peculiar latent period of 5 to 8 years.

HIV is a retrovirus, and retroviruses do not kill cells. On the contrary, they depend on living cells to reproduce. This is why retroviruses were the most plausible viral carcinogens in President Nixon's "War on Cancer". Paradoxically: the retrovirus called HIV is said to cause AIDS by killing T-cells. In fact, Robert Gallo and others have observed that T-cells in culture produce much more virus than is ever produced in AIDS patients, yet survive indefinitely, developing into immortal lines.

No known virus discriminates between men and women, or between heterosexuals and homosexuals. Paradoxically: even eight years into the epidemic, AIDS shows an absolute preference for men (92%).

The transfusion cases have been used as an argument for the HIV hypothesis, yet transfusions do not discriminate between HIV and all other microbes, toxins, etc. that are in the blood. That the transfusion argument is not strong, but tenuous, is shown by the control group of 14,000 hemophiliacs in the United States who are antibody positive, yet only 300 (2%) of whom have developed any of the many symptoms of AIDS. The low incidence is even more striking in light of the fact that hemophiliacs are a congenitally sickly population; only a few years ago, their average life expectancy was 11 years. Furthermore, it is now three years since the HIV antibody test came into use to screen blood. We should have seen at least a levelling off of the "transfusion cases", but contrary to expectations, they have just doubled.

According to basic logic, a virus or other pathogen would at least have to be present when it causes disease. This is Koch's first postulate for identifying a causative pathogen, which states that the presumed causative agent must be present in all cases of the disease. However, HIV can only be isolated in 50% of AIDS cases. Although there are unpublished observations that the figure can be pushed up to 100%, this is not consistent with the fact that pro-viral DNA cannot be detected in a substantial proportion of AIDS cases. Gallo could only detect pro-viral DNA in 15% of AIDS cases. A recent article in Science reported being unable to detect pro-viral DNA in a significant number of AIDS cases, even using the most sensitive techniques.

Duesberg posed the question, why is the "AIDS virus" hypothesis so popular, in the face of so many paradoxes? He suggested that this was due to two problems in the field:

One: Progress in biological thought has not kept up with the rapid progress in technology. Only ten years ago, scientists would never have detected a latent virus that is only active in one out of every 100,000 T-cells.

With their limited tools, Koch or Pasteur or Enders or Sabin were forced to look for microbes at clinically relevant titers. Indeed, Koch's first postulate needs to be amended now, in light of the technology of the present, to state that pathogens must not only be detectable, by the most sensitive techniques available, but must also be biochemically active in more cells than the host can spare or regenerate.

Two: AIDS is a <u>syndrome</u>, not a single infectious disease. The spectrum of diseases is truly impressive... yet such things as lymphoma and Kaposi's sarcoma cannot be attributed to immune deficiency, as is shown by the example of the nude mice. Nor does immune deficiency explain dementia.

In short, the one-virus, one-disease concept is hard to reconcile with the AIDS situation, although people would like to see it that way. AIDS propaganda has transformed a latent, non-cytocidal retrovirus, a "Sleeping Beauty", into a vicious killer virus. AIDS propaganda has reduced a complex syndrome to a single disease entity with a single cause. What we need to do is look at "risk behavior", which may hold the keys to the many diseases of AIDS.

Anthony Fauci

Anthony Fauci, Director of the National Institute of Allergy and Infectious Diseases (NIAID), has become the most publicly prominent member of the "AIDS establishment", often quoted in the press and featured on television shows. His presentation, while aspiring to be a point-by-point rebuttal to Duesberg, consisted mainly of disconnected assertions, delivered in a tone of petulant indignation. Epidemiological studies conducted in San Francisco and unpublished laboratory reports seemed to be the basis of most of his statements. So far as I could tell, he understood virtually none of Duesberg's arguments; whatever else Fauci may be, he is not a philosopher.

It is not true, Fauci said, that HIV is inactive; sometimes there are "bursts of activity". It is false to say that nothing is happening: HIV is "insidiously destroying the immune system" in asymptomatic but infected people.

The AIDS virus is unique in that its major target is the immune system itself. The disease is not HIV infection; "it is the opportunistic infections and neoplasms that kill the individual." Auto-immune phenomena, etc. can also be taken into account, in addition to the direct cytocidal effect, which is clearly demonstrated in vitro. The macrophages can serve as a reservoir, where the virus can hide out without being detected by the immune system.

According to Duesberg, if you're infected this means, "hurrah, your body has won!" This flies negatively in the face of the data, that within five years, 90% of seropositive individuals will have deleterious effects on their immune system [based on an unpublished San Francisco study].

Fauci countered Duesberg's point on "discrimination" by saying that the point was the mechanism of transmission. Risk behavior simply meant coming into contact with the virus. He then asked a series of abusively rhetorical questions: "What kind of risk behavior", he demanded, "does the infant born of an infected mother have?" "And what about the 50-year-old woman who received a blood transfusion from an infected donor?" (The answer to the first question is: 1) in the decade of the AIDS epidemic, there have been only a few hundred reported cases of infants with AIDS, 2) infants are not yet immunocompetent, and 3) virtually all infants with AIDS were born to mothers who were drug abusers -- as everyone ought to know, drugs cause birth defects. The answer to the second question is that a 50-year old woman who requires a blood transfusion is already at risk, and that blood transfusions involve massive exposure to microbes and toxins of all kinds.)

Fauci addressed the question of Koch's first postulate by asserting that "good labs" could find the virus in 90-95% of the cases -- that it was too much to expect 100%, because any technique has a limitation. He concluded by saying, "The data strongly, if not overwhelming, indicates [sic] that HIV is the cause of AIDS." (This is a step backward -- only a few weeks ago, Fauci found the evidence "overwhelming".)

In the question period, Beluda asked if the evidence were sufficient that HIV is necessary for the development of AIDS. Fauci replied that he hoped the epidemiologists would answer that question.

William Haseltine

William Haseltine, Chief of the Laboratory of Biochemical Pharmacology at the Dana Farber Cancer Center of Harvard Medical School, appeared to be an angry man. His presentation was devoted largely to personal attacks on Duesberg, in a manner which two of my colleagues described as "brutal" and "vicious". Haseltine's anger can probably be attributed to Celia Farber's interview with Duesberg in SPIN (January 1988), in which Duesberg stated:

> William Haseltine and Max Essex, who are two of the top five AIDS researchers in the country, have millions in stocks in a company they founded that has developed and will sell AIDS kits that test for HIV. How could they be objective?

When Celia Farber contacted Haseltine, he confirmed his and Essex's business arrangement with Cambridge Bio-Science, a company that sells HIV testing kits. Said Haseltine: "I deeply resent the implication that my business investments have affected my work."[5]

---

[5]Celia Farber, (interview with Duesberg) "a.i.d.s.: Words From the Front", SPIN, January 1988.

Haseltine accused Duesberg of "serious confusion and misrepresentation of fact". He said that when rational arguments don't hold up, Duesberg "has resorted to personal attack; he has impugned the motivations of individuals and institutions."

Haseltine asserted that "HIV is demonstrably cytopathic", though he didn't say how.

He quoted Duesberg as having said that antibodies were "good news". Not so, said Haseltine, to be antibody positive is very bad news for the health of the individual.

Haseltine said it was not true that there was no detectable viremia in AIDS patients, and said he would show a slide "with the current perception with regard to viremia...during the later course of infection, one sees rising antigenemia in most persons infected."

He attacked Duesberg's "paradox", that the AIDS virus seemed to be able to discriminate between boys and girls, by saying that this was not true outside the U.S. -- in Africa, about equal numbers of men and women develop AIDS. (He seemed oblivious to the paradox that a microbe should be able to discriminate in one country, but not in another.)

According to Haseltine, Rubin and Duesberg were confused about nude mice, which in certain classes were capable of "mounting a vigorous immune response".

The most dramatic moment in the forum came when Haseltine began showing his slides; it deserves a separate section:

Haseltine's Fake Slide

In presenting his first slide, Haseltine said:

This gives us a summary of the virology. Dr. Duesberg asserts that during the later phases of the disease one does not see free virus in circulation. That is not generally reflected in the patients. During the latter phase of the disease, the black line represents either virus titer or viral antigens directly detectable in the circulation. It rises later in the disease. That rise is concomitant with the period when T-cells fall. So it is not the case, the central assertion he has made in his arguments, that one does not have viremia.

At this point Duesberg asked, "Why are there no units on that slide?" Haseltine's response was, "Don't interrupt me; I didn't interrupt you." Duesberg replied, "I merely asked why the slide has no units on it." Haseltine angrily refused to answer the question, and the chairman intervened, saying that questions would have to wait until the presentation was finished.

Perhaps Duesberg ought to have waited, but one can understand his impatience. Witnessing a fast-flowing stream of propaganda, he spotted something that was obviously wrong, and wanted to confront it before the moment was lost. That his suspicions were more than justified became clear later.

In the question period following Haseltine's presentation, Harry Rubin asked Haseltine if he could provide a reference for his statement that nude mice were capable of mounting a vigorous immune response. Haseltine said that there was a large literature on nude mice: "If you haven't read it, how can I discuss it with you?". Rubin gently replied that perhaps he had, but that he had only asked for a reference.

Duesberg then requested that the slide be shown on the screen again, and asked if it were an accident that the slide had no units on it. (See photograph of slide. The vertical axes have no units, and the chronological notations on the horizontal axis are gibberish.) Haseltine was unable to answer the question himself, and asked Dr. Robert Redfield of the Walter Reed Army Research Institute, sitting in the audience, to explain how the slide was prepared. Redfield said something to the effect that "different measurements were used", a grossly inadequate explanation. When Duesberg persisted, Haseltine became truculent, and said that Duesberg should read the literature, because there were

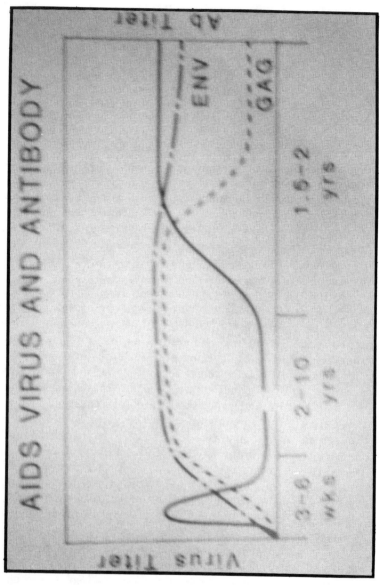

The fake slide. No units on the y axes and gibberish on the x axis.

different measures that could be used. With no satisfactory answer forthcoming, the chairman moved on.

The truth about the Slide Without Units came out
in the evening, at a party at the home of Dr. Harris
Coulter (author of AIDS and Syphilis: The Hidden
Link). In a relaxed and convivial mood, Redfield
admitted, in the presence of Duesberg, Rubin, myself,
and several other witnesses, that the graph had been
prepared to illustrate a theoretical possibility. It had
no units on it for the simple reason that it was not
based on any data at all. In other words, the slide
was a fake.

It is difficult to think of an innocent explanation
for Haseltine's behavior. If he didn't know what the
slide meant, or whether or not it was real, then he
shouldn't have used it. Haseltine presented the slide
as though it represented scientific findings, whereas it
really represented speculation. It is not unfair to call
this kind of misrepresentation, fraud. Nor is it making
too much out of one fake slide. If someone will cheat
in little things, he will cheat in big things as well. In
my book, Haseltine has forfeited his claim to scientific
credibility.

Warren Winkelstein

Warren Winkelstein, Professor of Biomedical and
Environmental Health Sciences, School of Public Health,
University of California at Berkeley, gave a talk entitled "Epidemiological Observations on the Causal
Nature of the Association Between Infection by the
Human Immunodeficiency Virus and the Acquired Immunodeficiency Syndrome". He was the only panelist
to provide printed copies of his talk, something much
appreciated by us journalists.

Briefly, the point of Winkelstein's presentation is
that Koch's postulates should be superseded by new
standards for establishing the causal relationship
between microbes and disease, and that these standards

should be based upon "epidemiology", or, as it were, correlations of various kinds.

Winkelstein and colleagues in San Francisco, under the auspices of Fauci's National Institute of Allergy and Infectious Diseases, studied a sample of single men, 25-54 years of age, over a period of three and a half years. Data were collected on HIV antibody status over time, on progression to AIDS, and on various other clinical parameters.

They found that none of the heterosexual males and none of the gay men who remained seronegative developed AIDS, whereas 13% of the men who were seropositive upon entry into the study, and 8% of those who became positive during the course of the study developed AIDS. Further, they found that a progressive decline in T-4 cells occurred among those who were seropositive.

They concluded that epidemiological data from their study, together with data from a related San Francisco study (conducted among a cohort of gay men recruited from VD clinics in 1978 for a hepatitis B study), supported "the hypothesis of a causal association between HIV infection and AIDS."

All in all, a grim scenario, according to which testing positive for HIV antibodies would truly be a "prognosis for death". I am skeptical, but as a survey research professional I reserve the right to withhold judgment until I have seen full reports on both San Francisco studies. At minimum such reports would have to include full descriptions of methodology; all questionnaires, recording forms, and field materials; sampling procedures; and computer tabulations.

At any rate, I do not accept the proposition that Koch's postulates should be abandoned in favor of epidemiological correlations. This would be a step backward, a step away from scientific rigor, a stop towards impressionism and confusion.

Murray Gardner

Murray Gardner, Chairman of the Department of Pathology, University of California at Davis, spoke about lentiviruses and animals. The man is apparently a failed standup comedian. During his presentation he danced back and forth behind the table, gesturing wildly, urging the audience to laugh along with him at the absurdity of doubting, even for a moment, that HIV was the cause of AIDS. We were told that the animals had "little understanding of co-factors", that their diseases had "nothing to do with lifestyle", and so on. Gardner had begun his clown act even earlier, making faces during Rubin's presentation.

Virtually nothing Gardner said was relevant, and little was memorable, except perhaps a few mistakes. A slide of his referred to the "pathogenicity of new HIV strains, e.g., HIV-2". This is wrong: HIV-1 and HIV-2 are not different strains of each other; they are completely different viruses; they differ in genetic structure by up to 60%; they do not have a closely-related common ancestor.

On this basis Dr. Joseph Sonnabend in New York City has formulated an "evolutionary argument" against the HIV hypothesis, which runs roughly as follows: There is no longer just one "AIDS virus"; there are several, perhaps as many as four or five at last count. It is now claimed that both HIV-1 and HIV-2 are capable of causing AIDS, a disease which allegedly appeared in the world for the first time only a few years ago. However, viruses are products of evolution, and very ancient -- there is no such thing as a "new" virus. The proposition that, within the space of a few years, two different viruses, each capable of causing the same new disease, should have come into being, or should have gone from an animal reservoir to susceptible human populations, is beyond the bounds of probability.

Gardner concluded his presentation by winking at the audience. It reminded me of one critic's comment on a cheaply made horror movie, that the zombies were less frightening than the attempts at humor.

Roger Detels

Roger Detels, Professor of Public Health, University of California at Los Angeles, began his talk by saying that it was good to continue questioning judgments. In context, this amounted to an apology to Duesberg and Rubin for the rudeness with which they had been treated. It was a gracious gesture on his part.

Detels discussed the San Francisco "Multi-Center AIDS Cohort Study", in which an annual "attack rate" of 5% was found among the seropositive gay men studied. That is, each year 5% of the seropositives came down with AIDS. (Harry Rubin was to point out later, that if 1-3 million Americans are seropositive, according to CDC estimates, and if the annual attack rate is 5%, simple arithmetic indicates that every year 50,000 to 150,000 people ought to develop AIDS.)

During the question period, pathogenesis was mentioned again, and Haseltine entered the fray, insisting that there were plenty of mechanisms that could explain pathogenesis, and that it was not necessary to discuss it.

Questions From The Audience

The first audience participant was Harvey Bialy, Research Editor of Bio/Technology. His remarks can be found in more detail in an editorial in the February issue of Bio/Technology[6]. The gist is that several recent articles have cited antigenemia findings to suggest that HIV may, after all, be active during the fatal, late stages of AIDS. However, the papers contain serious mathematical and other discrepancies. Bialy maintained that it was the responsibility of

---

[6]Harvey Bialy, "Commentary: Where is the Virus? And Where is the Press?", Bio/Technology, February 1988.

scientists, as well as journalists, to look at data critically and ask the hard questions.

The second speaker from the audience was Dr. Harris Coulter, who asked whether findings from the San Francisco City Clinic study, based on a sample of gay men who had hepatitis B, and who were highly promiscuous and heavily into recreational drugs, could be extrapolated to all of the people in the U.S. who were seropositive. The epidemiologists were either unable or unwilling to answer his question. Coulter persisted, asking the question in several different ways, each of which was perfectly clear. But the "AIDS experts" could not respond. This was truly amazing, for the question was one of the most basic in all of statistics: How representative is a sample of a particular universe? Can one project findings from the sample to the target universe?

Next Dr. Nathaniel Lehrman spoke, emphasizing the need to re-examine the etiology of AIDS, not only because of the questions raised by Duesberg and others, but because its epidemiology is far more consistent with a toxic illness than with an infectious one. How could AIDS be only an infection, and spreading so rapidly, when, according to Surgeon General C. Everett Koop, M.D., not one of 750 accidental inoculees with the blood or body fluids of known AIDS patients developed the disease, and only three then developed antibodies to HIV?

Chemical causes of immune deficiency, stated Lehrman, have long been known, and one group of chemicals, known to produce immune suppression, may be a cause of AIDS in the homosexual community: inhaled nitrites, or "poppers". Could other chemicals also be involved in producing immune suppression and AIDS? Lehrman concluded by saying that the possibility that chemical toxicity plays a significant causal role in AIDS ought to be investigated, and that additional methods in diagnosing, treating and researching the syndrome should be adopted. One such step would be spectrophotometric and similar investigation of AIDS patients for unusual, immune-suppressive substances within their bodies.

I spoke next, and said it was high time that those who advanced the hypothesis that HIV was the cause of AIDS should publish a monograph in an appropriate journal, which would bring together all the evidence supporting their hypothesis, which would take into account the critiques made by Duesberg and others, and which would contain proper references for all assertions made. Then I said that the epidemiological research on AIDS had been very poor, completely unacceptable by the standards of professional survey research. Ever since 1984, Public Health Service surveys have concentrated only on such things as "modes of transmission", or "risk factors for seroconversion", as a result of which we know almost nothing about the characteristics of PWAs. We have no idea what the IV drug users with AIDS are like, other than the "risk group" label that has been slapped on them. Finally, I said it was disgraceful that AZT was still being marketed, a poisonous drug without a single scientifically-established benefit. When would the AIDS establishment admit that the AZT trials, on which approval of the drug was based, were fraudulent?[7]

Finally, Michael Specter, a reporter from the Washington Post, demanded that Duesberg give him a yes or no answer to the question, "Do you still maintain that someone should be overjoyed to find out he is positive?" When Duesberg paused, the way one does when confronted with an obstreperous barbarian, Specter started yelling, "Answer the question! Yes or No? Why won't you answer the question?" Duesberg, when he got a chance, replied that he would answer the question, but in his own words, not Specter's. The nuances of his answer were not appreciated.

---

[7]Native Issues 235 and 258.

Summing Up

For the debate on the cause(s) of AIDS to move forward, a number of questions of fact must be resolved, with proper references given for all assertions: Does HIV kill cells in vivo? If so, how? Is HIV really "more complex in its genetic makeup than any other known retrovirus" (as asserted in AmFAR's "Review of Operations: 1985-1986")? From what percentage of PWAs can HIV be isolated? From what percentage of PWAs can pro-viral DNA be detected? What is the definition of a "good lab"? Is viremia found in PWAs? If so, what virus titers are obtained, when, how, etc.? Are there (as asserted by Gallo et al.) both pathogenic and non-pathogenic strains of HIV? If so, how do they differ? Can "nude mice" really mount a vigorous immune response (as asserted by Haseltine)? Is a full report available on the epidemiological research conducted in San Francisco?

The forum exposed the bankruptcy of the arguments used by the HIV advocates. Only a few weeks ago they were trotting out at least half a dozen speculative mechanisms to explain how HIV <u>might</u> cause AIDS; during the forum, such speculations were abandoned, and the official line was, "We don't need to explain pathogenesis." The "AIDS virus" crowd cannot agree on even the most crucial questions of fact, as indicated above. At one moment HIV is ferociously killing T-cells; the next moment, "AIDS experts" are desperately scrounging around for "indirect mechanisms". "Epidemiology" has been called in as a last ditch effort to rescue the HIV hypothesis, and yet the epidemiology conducted by the AIDS establishment to date has been quite bad, totally unacceptable by the standards of professional survey research (of which "epidemiology" is a subspecies). While the San Francisco studies may "strongly support" the HIV hypothesis, they could not prove it, even if the data were correct (and this cannot be determined until a proper report is issued), because there remain alternative explanations to account for the correlation between HIV antibodies and AIDS — namely, that HIV is itself an opportunistic infection in the AID Syndrome, that HIV is a marker for AIDS.

I am more convinced than ever that HIV is not the cause of AIDS. If the HIV advocates were sure of their hypothesis, they would want to enlighten Duesberg and the rest of us; they would want to publish their arguments in a proper scientific journal, complete with references. They would not need to resort to stonewalling, deception, and personal abuse.

#

XIII. Excerpt From Interview with Peter Duesberg
25 March 1990

Following is an excerpt from an interview that took place in New York City on 25 March 1990. At a forum the previous evening Duesberg had presented his "Risk-AIDS" hypothesis, which he has formulated as an alternative to the prevailing "HIV-AIDS" hypothesis.[1]

The "Risk-AIDS" hypothesis recognizes that "AIDS" is officially defined by the CDC as any of over two dozen old diseases in the presence of antibodies to HIV, a probably harmless retrovirus. It suggests that different "risk groups" and different individuals may be getting sick in different ways and for different reasons. We should examine the risks that impinge on them. There may be very good and even obvious reasons why intravenous drug users, a very small subset of gay men, a very small percentage of hemophiliacs, a minuscule number of transfusion recipients, and a minuscule number of children have gotten sick in ways that qualified for a diagnosis of "AIDS".

John Lauritsen: We should be open-minded, but somehow drugs make sense to me [as a cause of AIDS].

Peter Duesberg: It's better than that. We have 30% confirmed IV drug users, recorded by the CDC. That's a very solid link. They are injecting heroin, probably on a daily basis, in millimolar amounts. To ignore that, or not to consider that, as a factor of direct or indirect immune suppression, is at least negligent from a chemical point of view.

---

[1] See Peter Duesberg; "AIDS: Non-Infectious Deficiencies Acquired By Drug Consumption And Other Risk Factors"; Research in Immunology; 1990, 141 (in press).

JL: or schizophrenic.

PD: And AZT — we don't need to ask any further. It was awarded the Nobel prize for killing cells.

JL: This brings up another thing. The AIDS epidemic appears to have peaked already, probably about in the second part of 1988.[2] But if 50,000 or more people with HIV antibodies are taking AZT, then there may be another upswing in incidence, if these people end up being listed as "AIDS cases".

PD: They will have to be. Clearly. They will be perfect AIDS cases. Their immune systems will be intoxicated by AZT and they will be antibody positive. That's the definition of an AIDS case.

JL: Right. And yet it would really be AZT poisoning. Now, let's talk about AZT. They've begun giving it to perhaps tens of thousands of people who are healthy but have HIV antibodies. What's the prognosis going to be for them.

PD: I do not see how they could possibly survive it, in the long run. So the prognosis is clear — either a fast or a slow death of the immune system, or death altogether, because all growing cells will be killed by incorporation of AZT. AZT is a DNA chain terminator. That's what it was designed for. So I don't think anybody could sustain that for a very long time. Variations may exist in the ability of individuals to take it up, because AZT, in order to get into the cells, needs to be phosphorylated, and that is done by enzymes that are called kinases — and people apparently differ with regard to kinases — at least cells in cul-

---

[2] See John Lauritsen, "Debate Over AIDS Incidence", Native Issue 363.

ture do and animals do, and likely people do too. And those who have less kinases won't take AZT up well. They'll essentially piss it out -- luckily. They would be more resistant. And others, who do take AZT up well, would be more sensitive and would be intoxicated much more effectively and much more directly.

JL: A DNA chain terminator -- what are the consequences of this?

PD: It's embarrassingly clear. It is simply stopping the growth of DNA. And you have to complete DNA cell synthesis. Cell division is based on doubling DNA, which is the central molecule of life. It contains all the genetic information. If you don't complete that, the cell is not viable. It will die. The information about an organism is written down in a code that we call DNA, the chromosome or nucleic acid. If that book isn't completely written, you are incomplete, you are not viable. You can only live if everything that is needed for a primate is in every single cell of your body -- that makes you John Lauritsen. If only half a copy is there, then you are no longer John Lauritsen. Then there is only half a cell, and most likely that cell will be dead, because it lacks important things that it needs for its survival.

JL: So basically, the very nature of AZT is to terminate life? Is that too strong?

PD: No. To terminate living cells. And of course to terminate life is a secondary consequence. The primary target is to kill all cells that are in the process of dividing. That what AZT was developed for, to kill cancer cells. And as we all know, chemotherapy is aimed at growing cells. The benefit is that we kill the tumor cells. The heavy price we pay in all chemotherapy is that all normal cells growing at the time will also be killed. Fortunately, you can often regenerate the normal cells, and if you are lucky, the tumor will not be regenerated. In reality though, you often get a remission. The tumor will be reduced to a small number of cells, and then will come back. And then the patient needs a second round of chemotherapy. But the principle is to kill everything that's growing at the time, and hope you wipe out the enemy better than your friends.

JL: I thought that chemotherapy was usually given for a relatively short period of time.

PD: It is. You couldn't sustain it any longer. You hope to wipe out the tumor in that short time, and hope for the patient to regenerate.

JL: And yet AZT, a form of chemotherapy, is being given now, on a 24-hour basis, with the idea that people will take it as long as they live.

PD: Yes -- that is simply incomprehensible to me. I cannot come up with a rational explanation. I haven't heard one. In fact, they always avoid one-- they keep saying it has been shown empirically to prolong life. That is very difficult for me to accept. I'm trying to take the data for what they are, and to criticize them on the basis of intrinsic inconsistencies, but this one I simply can't accept. I cannot see how DNA chain termination could prolong life, DNA being the basis of life. How DNA chain termination could prolong life is very difficult for me to understand, in fact, impossible.

JL: I agree, and we know that the Phase II trials were fraudulent. There's no nice way to put it: they were fraudulent. And so, not only is the theory behind AZT wrong, but the "findings" supporting it are phoney as well.

#

XIV. Incompetence In AIDS Epidemiology
Speech To Forum On Causes Of AIDS
Bronx Community College, 16 December 1988

In the discourse on "AIDS", the word, "epidemiology", is used a great deal. Although the word is not clearly defined, most epidemiology consists of what I would call "survey research". This is my field, one in which I have two decades of experience. And so I am on home ground in criticizing epidemiological research done by the Centers for Disease Control (CDC) and other branches of the Public Health Service (PHS).

Those of you who are following the debate over whether HIV is the cause of "AIDS" have probably read -- or ought to read -- the debate that appeared in the 29 July 1989 issue of Science. In that issue, Peter Duesberg argued that "HIV Is Not the Cause of AIDS", and he was opposed by William Blattner, Robert Gallo, and Howard Temin, who argued that "HIV Causes AIDS". Each side was permitted a rebuttal. In the decade that the "AIDS epidemic" has been with us, this is the only time that members of the "AIDS establishment" have condescended to defend the HIV hypothesis in open debate. And Gallo & Co. lost, in no uncertain terms. They did not even attempt to respond to Duesberg's main arguments, and had to fall back upon ad hominem attacks and flimsy appeals to "epidemiology". In his rebuttal Duesberg stated that epidemiology was not sufficient to prove that HIV was the cause of "AIDS", that correlation is not the same as causation.

This is correct, and one of the first things a student learns in studying statistics: Correlation implies, but does not prove causation. Even if there is a strong correlation between two or more things, it is still necessary to dig in and prove, by whatever means are appropriate, that the relationship is one of cause and effect.

I'm going to go one step further and argue that, not only is epidemiology not sufficient to prove that HIV causes "AIDS", but that the epidemiology -- or survey research, as it were -- done by government "scientists" is very bad. Their work has been far below the standards of professional survey research. I sometimes brood over whether their shortcomings are due to dishonesty or to incompetence, and conclude-- both! They are dishonest and they are incompetent. And their incompetence stretches all the way from the CDC, whose periodic reports of surveillance information reveal that they are unaware of the most elementary statistical conventions, to the New York City Health Department, which (despite several Ph.D.'s in their ranks) have not yet mastered grade school arithmetic.

From the very beginning, the Public Health Service was determined to construct "AIDS" as a new disease caused by a new infectious agent. According to the official paradigm, "AIDS" is a single disease entity with a single cause, which is an infectious agent, which is a newly discovered retrovirus now known as HIV-1. In fact, not a single one of these propositions has been established scientifically. Not one of the two dozen diseases in the syndrome is new. Neither is immune deficiency new, and it is well known that the condition can have many causes, from chemicals, to malnutrition, to bad genes, to radiation, to old age. The prevailing "AIDS" paradigm consists of unsupported assumptions-- the products of dubious research, of a self-perpetuating delusional system, of endless reiteration in the popular and "scientific" literature.

I began to study the "AIDS" literature in 1983, being particularly impressed that "AIDS" was not behaving like an infectious disease. Over time, the proportions of "AIDS" cases accounted for by each of the "risk groups" remained almost constant.

I have analyzed the proportions of "AIDS" cases accounted for by each of the "risk groups" at two points in time: as of December 1984 and then more

than five years later, as of February 1990.[1] In these
five years the number of "AIDS" cases increased more
than fifteen-fold (from 7609 in 1984 to 117,781 in
1990), and yet the proportions of the various risk
groups remain virtually identical. It is clear that
"AIDS" is compartmentalized, confined almost entirely
to two main groups: gay men and intravenous drug
users (IVDUs). This is the central epidemiological
puzzle of "AIDS", and it must be explained. If "AIDS"
is really an infectious disease, why is it not spreading?
The compartmentalization of "AIDS" strongly suggests
that environmental (or "lifestyle") factors play a role
in causing the syndrome, either as primary causes or
as "co-factors".

It became apparent as early as 1984 that the epidemiology of "AIDS" was more consistent with a toxicological model than with an infectious disease model.
I began to focus upon the very heavy "recreational
drug" use found among certain subsets of gay men, and
in particular upon one drug: "poppers" or nitrite inhalants. The use of this drug has been confined
almost entirely to gay men. All of you in the audience
who are gay men know what poppers are. The rest of
you have probably never heard of them. I'll explain.

Poppers are little bottles containing a liquid mixture
of isobutyl nitrite and other chemicals. When inhaled
just before orgasm, poppers seem to enhance and
prolong the sensation. Poppers facilitate anal intercourse by relaxing the muscles in the rectum and
deadening the sense of pain. They are addictive, at
least psychologically, and some gay men have been
known to snort them around the clock. Some "AIDS
patients", in New York and San Francisco, had popper
bottles on the table by their death bed; they continued
to inhale them as long as they could breathe.

---

[1]I have updated the data and the graph for this
book.

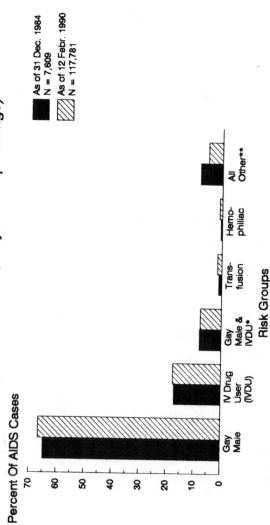

TOTAL UNITED STATES AIDS CASES
By Risk Group
1984 - 1990

Risk Group Proportions Have Hardly Changed In Five Years!
(If AIDS Is Infectious, Why Isn't It Spreading?)

Percent Of AIDS Cases

■ As of 31 Dec. 1984
N = 7,609

▨ As of 12 Febr. 1990
N = 117,781

Risk Groups

Gay Male · IV Drug User (IVDU) · Gay Male & IVDU* · Trans-fusion · Hemo-philiac · All Other**

*Until 1985 the CDC counted these only as "homo/bisexual men".
**Includes Haitians, "heterosexual contact", pediatric, and "other/unknown".

Graph by John Lauritsen

The Food and Drug Administration (FDA) has repeatedly refused to regulate poppers, giving the excuse that every bottle of poppers was labelled either "room odorizer" or "incense".   Now, there is no evidence that anyone ever used poppers as "incense", and the most parsimonious explanation for the FDA's "hands-off" policy would be bribery; the FDA has for many decades been a notoriously corrupt agency.[2]

I have collaborated since 1983 with Hank Wilson, a gay activist in San Francisco, who in 1981 founded the Committee to Monitor the Effects of Poppers.   In 1986 we published a book together (Death Rush: Poppers & AIDS), in an attempt to alert gay men to the dangers of poppers.

A summary of the medical case against poppers: Poppers are immunosuppressive.   They cause anemia, lung damage, serious skin burns, and death or brain damage from cardiovascular collapse or stroke.   Poppers cause genes to mutate and have the potential to cause cancer by producing deadly N-nitroso compounds. Poppers have been used successfully to commit suicide (by drinking) and murder (victim gagged with sock soaked with poppers).   There are strong epidemiological links between the use of poppers and the development of AIDS, and especially Kaposi's sarcoma (KS).   A six-

---

[2] See Morton Mintz, By Prescription Only (A report on the United States Food and Drug Administration, the American Medical Association, pharmaceutical manufacturers, and others in connection with the irrational and massive use of prescription drugs that may be worthless, injurious, or even lethal), Boston, 1967.

James S. Turner, The Chemical Feast: The Ralph Nader Study Group Report on Food Protection and the Food and Drug Administration, New York, 1970.

fold decrease in the incidence of KS over the past five years parallels a sharp decline in the use of poppers.

Obviously poppers are not the cause of "AIDS", since they were not used by the non-homosexual "AIDS" cases.   However, the drug is clearly hazardous to the health and high on the list of probable co-factors for causing "AIDS".

Although there is a very powerful connection between "AIDS" and drugs, the CDC has consistently obscured the connection.   For several years the CDC presented its surveillance statistics using a so-called "hierarchical presentation".   They listed the largest "risk category" first: homosexual/bisexual men.   Then they listed the next largest category, intravenous drug users (IVDUs), but they counted people here only if they had not already been counted in the first category.   What this did was to submerge the overlap group: IVDUs who were also gay men; these were counted as "homosexual/bisexual men", but not as IVDUs.   As a result of this statistical obscurantism, the CDC's tables showed IVDUs as comprising only about 17% of the "AIDS" cases, whereas in fact they comprised at least 25%.   The CDC finally abandoned this form of statistical trickery after an article of mine exposing it was published in half a dozen gay newspapers.[3]

In light of the compartmentalization of "AIDS", it is reasonable to hypothesize that the drugs used by IVDUs made them sick, either as sole cause or as contributing co-factor.   However, the government has done everything it can to suppress this hypothesis.

The official line is that "AIDS" is caused solely by an infectious agent, HIV-1, and that IV drug users became "infected" by sharing needles.   Unfortunately

---

[3] John Lauritsen, "CDC's Tables Obscure AIDS/-Drugs Connection", Philadelphia Gay News, 14 February 1985.

for this hypothesis, there is no evidence that all, or even most, IVDUs with "AIDS" ever did share needles. It has simply been assumed, but the research has never been done to verify the assumption.   To be sure, we know that some IVDUs do share needles.   But we also know that many IVDUs have never shared needles, and for very good reasons.   For many decades they have been well aware of the dangers of getting such deadly diseases as serum hepatitis this way.   And besides, why should they share needles?   An addict with a $60 a day habit can certainly afford a one-time purchase of $2 for a needle.   The research to determine whether or not all IV drug users with "AIDS" actually had shared needles would be simple, straightforward, and inexpensive, and it is incomprehensible why such research has not been done.

Heroin and other drugs injected by IVDUs are known to be immunosuppressive and otherwise dangerous.   It is blatantly probable that the drugs themselves (not shared needles) are the reason that IVDUs are developing "AIDS".   For many decades IVDUs have been dying of pneumonia.   This is nothing new.   Dr. Polly Thomas, of the New York City Health Department, has admitted that an IVDU with pneumonia and HIV antibodies would be counted as an "AIDS" case, with the assumption that HIV was the sole cause-- however, if the same IVDU had pneumonia but no HIV antibodies, it would be assumed that the drugs were the cause.   And yet there would be no difference in the clinical profiles: of the "AIDS-pneumonia" case or the "drugs-pneumonia" case.

It is amazing and deplorable that so many "AIDS" groups and public health departments have issued posters and brochures directed to IVDUs, telling in great detail how to sterilize needles.   The message is clear: continue shooting up drugs, but play it safe by sterilizing your needles.   (Drugs are safe, but needles are dangerous.)   This insanity is taking place in the midst of a so-called "War Against Drugs"!

By definition all of the IVDUs with "AIDS" were drug users. And yet, from the meager information we have, it is possible that nearly all of the gay men with "AIDS" were also drug users. Research ought to have been done years ago to find out the characteristics of people with "AIDS" (PWAs) within each of the risk groups. As it is, we know virtually nothing about the IVDU, transfusion, or hemophiliac cases, other than the "risk group" label that has been slapped on them.

A little information about gay men with "AIDS" comes from a study of the first 50 gay men with "AIDS", conducted by the CDC in 1982-1983.[4] In this study, the "AIDS" cases were compared with controls drawn from public venereal disease clinics and from private practices. The controls turned out to be almost complete clones of the cases, with one exception: they did not have "AIDS" -- yet. Nevertheless, the controls were far from healthy, and a number of them developed "AIDS" shortly after the study was completed.

Never in their report did the authors even attempt to explain what they had in mind when they designed their study, although they did admit that there was an inherent bias towards unity. In other words, the tendency would be falsely to overlook risk factors that were real. In their own words:

> The expected impact of these potential problems in control selection and classification would be to minimize differences between cases and controls rather than to create false differences.

The only significant difference that the investigators were able to identify between cases and con-

---

[4]Harold Jaffe et al., "National Case-Control Study of Kaposi's Sarcoma and Pneumocystis carinii Pneumonia in Homosexual Men: Part 1, Epidemiologic Results", Annals of Internal Medicine, August 1983.

trols concerned the number of sexual partners. The "AIDS" cases had had more sexual partners per year, although the controls had also been remarkably promiscuous. For several years this "finding" formed the sole basis of the government's risk reduction guidelines. They said, "To avoid getting AIDS, reduce your number of sexual partners." Surely this advice was inane.

Considering the fatal flaws in sample design and selection, analyses based on comparisons between the "AIDS" patients and the controls fall into the category of "garbage in, garbage out". The comparative data are worthless. However, the government researchers were wrong to plunge immediately into a comparative, case vs. control analysis. A professional analyst would first look at the data on the "AIDS" cases monadically (by themselves). When this is done, the findings are very interesting indeed.

When we look at the data on the "AIDS" cases monadically, we ask the questions, "What are these people like? What are their characteristics?" And the answer that comes out of this research is that these first 50 gay men with "AIDS" were highly promiscuous; that they had had many, many venereal diseases, over and over again; that they had been treated innumerable times with broad-spectrum antibiotics, powerful antiparasite drugs, etc.; and, perhaps most important, that they were heavy drug abusers.

The majority of these gay men with "AIDS" had used at least half a dozen different "recreational drugs", some of which are very dangerous. Nearly all of them were users of poppers, alcohol, and marijuana, and a majority were also users of amphetamines, cocaine, LSD and quaaludes. Other drugs frequently used were ethyl chloride, barbiturates, MDA, and phencyclidine. One-sixth of them were users of intravenous drugs, including heroin.

Looking at this profile, it is not surprising that these men got sick. Rather, it would have been amazing if any of them had remained healthy. There is only so much abuse that a body can take. These data ought immediately to have prompted an investigation into the role that recreational and medical drugs played in causing gay men to develop "AIDS". But no. The sole conclusion the government researchers reached was to tell gay men: "Reduce your number of sexual partners!"

Another example of bad survey research with dire consequences is a CDC study which predicted that 99% of those who were "seropositive" (i.e., who had antibodies to HIV-1) would go on to develop "AIDS". I've written an extensive exposé[5] of this study, so won't go into it now, except to say that I talked to the three authors of the study, and they agreed with me that their research did not support the "99%" conclusion. Nevertheless, the 99%-will-develop-"AIDS" nonsense is still being bandied about in the media, and is being used to scare perfectly healthy people into taking the poisonous drug, AZT.[6]

On the topic of AZT, I have copies here of the exposé I did on the FDA-conducted AZT trials, which were the basis of the drug's approval.[7] It would be inadequate merely to call the trials "invalid". They were fraudulent. This we know from documents that the FDA was forced to release under the Freedom of Information Act. Among many other kinds of sloppiness and misconduct, the federal investigators knowingly used data that they knew were false. And they gave two excuses for using false data. Excuse number one: if they didn't use the false data, they would have hardly any subjects left. And excuse number two: using the false data didn't really change the results

---

[5] Chapter III, "The Epidemiology of Fear".

[6] Native Issue 276.

[7] Chapter II, "AZT On Trial".

very much.   Needless to say, these are the excuses of fools and scoundrels.   No ethical scientist would ever knowingly use false data.

To sum up: at this point we don't know exactly what "AIDS" is, or what causes it.   We'd better find out.   All reasonable hypotheses ought to be investigated -- we've had too much premature closure, too many speculations that have ossified into dogma.   However, I believe that some day it will be established that "AIDS" is not a single disease entity, but rather divers conditions; that "AIDS" has multiple causes, of which the most important are chemicals (including medical and recreational drugs).   The truth will be known eventually.   For right now, we know more than enough to justify proclaiming an urgent warning to gay men, IV drug users, and others: Don't use drugs!   And don't take AZT!

#

APPENDIX: Articles by John Lauritsen from the New York Native

12-25 August 1985
Poppers and AIDS: The Scientific Overview

9-15 December 1985
The AIDS-Drugs Connection

Issue 184: 27 October 1986
Koch's Postulates Revisited: Another Look at the "AIDS Virus" Fiasco

Issue 203: 9 March 1987
Caveat Emptor: The Report of the National Academy of Sciences on AIDS Is Filled With Misinformation

Issue 215: 1 June 1987
First Things First: Some Thoughts on the "AIDS Virus" and AZT

Issue 220: 6 July 1987
Saying No To HIV: An Interview With Prof. Peter Duesberg, Who Says, "I Would Not Worry About Being Antibody Positive" (Reprinted, with corrections, in Christopher Street, Issue 118, December 1987)

Issue 235: 19 October 1987
AZT on Trial: Did the FDA Rush to Judgment-- And Thereby Further Endanger the Lives of Thousands of People?

Issue 240: 16 November 1987
Berkeley Backs Duesberg: Press Release Cites Two Articles Refuting HIV As the Cause of AIDS

Issue 243: 7 December 1987
Joseph Calls For Mandatory Testing: Prostitutes, Crackdowns on Commercial Sex Establishments on Health Commissioner's Agenda

Issue 246: 28 December 1987
AZT Update (also comment on Duesberg, <u>California Monthly</u> article)

Issue 250: 25 January 1988
The Amsterdam Conference

Issue 254: 22 February 1988
The HIV Debate

Issue 255: 29 February 1988
Non-Responses to Duesberg

Issue 258: 28 March 1988
AZT: Iatrogenic Genocide

Issue 263: 2 May 1988
The Racism Connection (A review of <u>AIDS, Africa and Racism</u> by Richard C. and Rosalind J. Chirimuuta)

Issue 264: 9 May 1988
Kangaroo Court Etiology: AmFAR Holds a Forum to Discredit Duesberg, But Winds Up Confirming Shabbiness of "Proof" of HIV as Sole Cause of AIDS

Issue 269: 6 June 1988
AZT Disinformation

Issue 273: 4 July 1988
Latex Lunacy

Issue 276: 1 August 1988
The Epidemiology of Fear

Issue 276: 1 August 1988
   Health Department Cuts "HIV Infection" Estimate In
   Half

Issue 281: 5 September 1988
   Incompetence As Usual

Issue 283: 19 September 1988
   More Sloppiness From the NYC Health Department

Issue 285: 3 October 1988
   Epidemiology in Graphics

Issue 286: 10 October 1988
   AIDS Incidence Dropping

Issue 298: 2 January 1989
   On The AZT Front: Part One

Issue 300: 16 January 1989
   On The AZT Front: Part Two

Issue 308: 13 March 1989
   Poppers: The End of an Era

Issue 317: 15 May 1989
   A Conference on Holistic Health

Issue 323: 26 June 1989
   Confusion in the HIV Ranks

Issue 323: 26 June 1989
   The First Gay Liberation Front Demonstration

Issue 331: 21 August 1989
   Science by Press Release

Issue 332: 28 August 1989
GMHC Announces Campaign To Encourage HIV Antibody Testing -- Adopts Major Policy Shift

Issue 340: 30 October 1989
AZT and Cancer

Issue 348: 18 December 1989
AZT Causes Cancer: Burroughs Wellcome Issues Advisory

Issue 354: 29 January 1990
U.S. Cuts AZT Dose in Half: Burroughs Wellcome Considering Recommending AZT for Symptomless HIV-Infected People

Issue 356: 12 February 1990
More Science by Press Conference: FDA Committee Recommends AZT For Healthy People

Issue 361: 19 March 1990
A "State of the Art" AZT Conference

Issue 363: 2 April 1990
Debate Over AIDS Incidence

Issue 367: 30 April 1990
AZT Watch: New Research Does Not Prove Efficacy

Index of Names

Altman, Lawrence 56

Arendt, Hannah 139

Ayers, Kenneth 134-135

Baltimore, David 131-132

Barry, David 17, 60, 76, 82, 84, 113

Beluda, Marcel 148, 151, 157

Bessen, Laura 101

Bialy, Harvey 130, 164-165

Blattner, William 58, 173

Broad, William 32

Broder, Samuel 19, 99, 102, 109

Callen, Michael 59, 60, 62, 68

Campbell, Duncan 102

Carpenter, Charles 126, 138

Casarett, Louis 98

Chernov, Harvey 12, 20, 44, 46, 94-98, 105, 107, 108

Chirimuuta, Richard and Rosalind 185

Coombs, Robert 131-132

Cooper, Ellen 14-15, 17, 20, 30, 32, 34, 43

Couch, Robert 137

Coulter, Harris 161, 165

Creagh-Kirk, Terri 22, 72, 76, 78-80, 85, 89

Darrow, William 49, 52-56

Deer, Brian 109, 125

Delaney, Martin 26, 65-66, 68-69

Detels, Roger 164

Diogenes 100-101

Douglas, Paul 69-70

Doull, John 98

Dournon, E. 130, 138

Duesberg, Peter 7-8, 10-12, 18, 25, 50-51, 58, 72-73, 99, 102, 112-113, 125, 131-132, 140-148, 152-158, 160-161, 164-166, 168-173, 184-185

Echenberg, Dean 55

Enders, John 155

Essex, Max 157

Farber, Celia 109, 125, 157

Fauci, Anthony 102-103, 137, 146-147, 151, 155-157, 161-162
Feinberg, Mark 131-132
Fischl, Margaret 13, 15, 17, 26-27, 32, 36, 64, 71, 102-103, 126-130, 133, 136-137
Friedland, Gerald 137
Gail, Mitchell 133-134
Gallo, Robert 58, 146, 153-154, 167, 173
Gardner, Murray 163-164
Garland, Judy 58
Gingell, Barry 60
Ginsberg, Harold 147, 148
Glenn, Frederick 62
Grossman, Ron 67-69
Hamilton, John 132-133
Haseltine, William 12, 73, 146-147, 151, 157-161, 164, 167
Hauptman, Lawrence 17, 30
Heckler, Margaret 143
Helbert, Matthew 101-102
Hellquist, Michael 121
Hilts, Philip 106, 110
Ho, David 131-132
Horwitz, Jerome 108-110
Jaffe, Harold 180
Jeremy 61
Joseph, Stephen 51, 185
Koch, Robert 144-145, 155, 157
Kolata, Gina 119
Krim, Mathilde 134
Lagakos, Stephen 128-130
Lambert, Bruce 51
Lange, Michael 66-69
Lehrman, Nat 165-166
Leishman, Katie 125
Lenin 125
Lui, Kung-Jong 49, 52-53, 55-56
Mason, James 51, 104-105, 110, 134
Mengele, Josef 99

Metroka, Craig 64
Mintz, Morton 177
Mitsuya, Hiroaki 99
Myers, Charles 99
Null, Gary 40, 125
Null, Steven 40
O'Loughlin, Ray 19
Pasteur, Louis 155
Peabody 100
Pinsky, Laura 64, 69-70
Pizzo, Philip 21, 130
Redfield, Robert 159, 161
Reger, Paul 50-51
Richman, Douglas 13-15, 17, 26-27, 32, 36, 64, 71,
    135-136
Rubin, Harry 146, 148-151, 158-161, 163-164
Rutherford, George 49, 52, 55-56
Sabin, Albert 155
Sanford, Jay 136-137
Schram, Neil 136-137
Scott 61
Shepperd, Alfred 115, 120
Smith, Peter 106
Sonnabend, Joseph 13, 65-69, 72, 88, 103, 125-126, 163
Specter, Michael 48-51, 53-54, 58, 143-144, 166
Staley, Peter 110
Stevens, Cladd 57
Sullivan, Louis 114, 123-124
Taub, Kenny 62-63
Temin, Howard 58, 173
Thomas, Polly 179
Turner, James 177
Varchoan, Robert 99
Volberding, Paul 128-130, 137
Wade, Nicholas 32
Weisburger, John 98
White, Ian 112
Wilson, Hank 24, 40, 177
Winkelstein, Warren 161-162

Wolfe, Sidney 94
Young, Frank 94
Young, Ian 125

Index of Subjects

ACTG Protocol 002 127-128
ACTG Protocol 016 90, 127
ACTG Protocol 019 89-92, 128-130
Aesop Fable 17
AIDS as non-infectious 165, 169, 174-175
AIDS as single disease entity, critique of concept 148-
      151, 155, 174, 183
AIDS cases, characteristics of 169, 181-182
AIDS Coalition To Unleash Power (ACT UP) 65-66, 88,
      110, 126
AIDS "risk group" analysis 169, 175-176, 178
American Foundation For AIDS Research (AmFAR)
      143, 167
Anecdotal reports, value of 20-22
Antiviral effect of AZT not proven 66-68
AZT as cause of AIDS 8, 10, 170
Business (Profits) 112-113, 115-116, 120-121
Cartesian reductionism 149
CD4 counts 135
Centers for Disease Control (CDC)
      Misleading statistics 178
      Case-control study 180-182
      Ignorance of statistical conventions 174
Chemotherapy, AZT as 7-8, 171-172
DNA chain termination 7-8, 170-171
Drug regulation in the U.S. 93-94
Drugs, recreational 23-24, 55-56, 165, 169, 175-183
Ethical issues 46-47, 66, 102-103, 139
Food and Drug Administration (FDA)
      Corruption in 40, 94, 177
      Cuts AZT Dose 114-116, 124
      Drug regulation 93-94
      Recommends AZT for healthy people 117-139
      Refusal to regulate poppers 40, 177

Gay Men's Health Crisis (GMHC) 70, 87
Genocide 10, 122
HIV hypothesis, critique of 7-8, 143-169
    Debate in Science 173
    Evolutionary argument against (Sonnabend) 163
"HIV infection" (antibodies), prognosis for 48-58, 161-
    162, 182
Intravenous drug users 169, 178-179
Kinases 170-171
Koch's Postulates 144-145, 157, 161-162
National Gay Rights Advocates (NGRA), law suit
    against NIH and FDA 19
National Institute of Allergies and Infectious Diseases
    (NIAID) 87, 90-91, 123-124, 127-128, 155
New York Blood Center Study 56-57
Nude mice studies 149, 155, 158, 160, 167
P-24 antigen test 18, 64, 67, 127, 130-132, 135, 164-
    165
People With AIDS Coalition (PWAC) 59-63
Phase II Trials 13-20, 25-47, 71, 88, 130, 139, 172
    Unblinding of 30-32, 66
Philosophy: AZT 22-23, 72-73
Philosophy: Recovery 23-24
Poppers (nitrite inhalants) 40, 175, 177-178, 181
Project Inform 26, 65, 87
Risk-AIDS hypothesis (Duesberg) 169
Stockholm abstracts 20-21, 68, 71
Survival Study 17, 22, 71-86, 88-89, 130
Toxicity of AZT 11-12, 20, 25, 44-46, 94-103, 114,
    118, 137, 170-172
    Anemia 44-46,
    Cancer, potential to cause 44, 94-100, 104-113, 115,
        118, 134-135, 138
    Chronic vs. acute 97-99, 115, 118-119, 137
    Muscular atrophy 100-102, 136-137
    Mutagenesis 95
Toxicologic model of AIDS causation 169-170, 175, 183
Venereal diseases 55, 180-181
Veterans Administration Study #298 131-132